Path Notes
of an American
Ninja Master

Path Notes
of an American
Ninja Master

by
Glenn J. Morris, Ph.D.,
D.Sc., Oshihan
Shidoshi in Togakure Ryu Bujinkan Ninpo

North Atlantic Books
Berkeley, California

Path Notes of an American Ninja Master

Copyright © 1993 Glenn J. Morris, Ph.D. All rights reserved. No part of this publication may be reproduced or transmitted in any form or by any means, electronic or mechanical, including photocopy, or any information storage or retrieval system, without written permission of the publisher. Printed in the United States of America.

Published by
North Atlantic Books
P.O. Box 12327
Berkeley, California 94701

Cover and book design by Paula Morrison
Typeset by Catherine Campaigne

Path Notes of an American Ninja Master is sponsored by The Society for the Study of Native Arts and Sciences, a nonprofit educational corporation whose goals are to develop an educational and cross-cultural perspective linking various scientific, social and artistic fields; to nurture a holistic view of arts, sciences, humanities, and healing; and to publish and distribute literature on the relationship of mind, body and nature.

Library of Congress Cataloging-in-Publication Data
Morris, Glenn, 1944–
    Pathnotes of an American ninja master / Glenn Morris.
      p. cm.
    Includes bibliographical references.
    ISBN 1-55643-157-0
    1. Ch'i kung.   I. Title.
RA781.8.M67 1993
796.8'15—dc20   93-8031
                                                      CIP

2 3 4 5 6 7 8 9 / 97 96 95 94

Table of Contents

Acknowledgments

This book is for my parents, my wives, and their children who became my own. It is for Linda who sent me away to follow my heart's desire and welcomed me home when I'd achieved a goal few would seek and fewer understand. It is dedicated to my students and friends who struggled with me as we all learned "the ways of strategy," and to those whose particular need for transformation draws them to the life-giving sword inherent in the highest levels of mastery in the martial arts, may they continue to fear no evil.

I would like to thank the following master teachers of Togakure Ryu Ninpo for their toleration of my eccentricities and for allowing me to become a part of their dream: Masaaki Hatsumi-Soke, thirty-fourth linear grandmaster of the Togakure Ryu, who brought the ninja out of the dark and took the risk of teaching *gaijin* (round-eyed devils); Stephen Hayes, who started the Ninja Boom in the United States; Bud and Bonnie Malmstrom, who are living examples of the loving heart; Kevin Millis of Shibu West, who sometimes shares his life and perspective; the Japanese *shihan*, Seno-san and Kan-san, for their continual sacrifice of their bodies in endless years of demos; Shiraishi-sensei and Ishizuka-sensei, for their lessons and hospitality when I was in their homes, training, or partying with them; Larry Turner and Greg Kowalski, who shared their expertise with me, and all the others who had the courage to look behind the propaganda, go to Japan, and become teachers of Bujinkan.

Other enlightened martial artists who contributed to my development include Shichidan Sherman Harrill of Carson City, Iowa, who is a magnificent teacher of Isshinryu Karate, and Leo Sebregst, who heads the Wu Shu Association of South Africa and whose teachings are available to all races in the city of Johannesburg.

John Yono, a boxer living in Livonia, Michigan, has provided interesting insights from a totally self-taught, no-respect-for-the-loser, Middle Eastern perspective.

Alternative medical systems have also played a necessary and positive role. The Chinese National Institute of Chi Kung in Moulton, Alabama, has a very good correspondence course for the development of *chi* (bioelectrical energy or subtle energy). Mantak Chia and Steven Chang have written extremely valuable works for those interested in working with their bodies' electrical systems.

Psychologists and healers who have chosen to be part of the Midwest Association of Humanistic Psychology have shared their knowledge and skills with me over the last ten years and provided a wonderful sounding board as well as confirmation that some of the rather strange phenomena I experienced were felt by others. Were it not for annual conventions where I could observe Trager enthusiasts, Reiki workers, and meditators of various ilk, as well as get on their tables, I feel I might have lost my sanity. Cynthia Raczko of Ann Arbor; Ilana Rubenfeld of Rubenfeld Synergy; Lisi Graves of Charlestown, Indiana; Treesa Weaver of Hillsdale, Michigan; and M. Cohen-Nehemia, founder of the Mitzvah Technique of Toronto, Canada, have wonderful skills in bodywork.

Denise Hillyard taught me many things about friendship across generations, and without the computer knowledge of Denise's Envoi Design in Cincinnati I'd never have been able to pull off this book. Dan Vettes at Jackson Community College MacLab helped me set up the book one frustrating afternoon.

Steve Noonkesser, Campbell Walker, Randall Reising, Cortney Strother, Toffesse Alemu, Suzanne Carlson, Kevin Brown, Skip Lepire, Rick Pinter, Karim abu Shakra of Jordan, Ted Consengco, Andy Tucker, Rick Groves, Dr. Richard Grant, L. J. Lavene, Shawn Phillips, Jaime Lombard, and Blake Poindexter all achieved the rank of *shodan* (first degree black belt) or higher in my self-protection course, *hoshinjutsu* (weapon heart skills) while completing their bachelor's degrees. They suffered my abuse, became my friends, and taught me what they wanted to learn. Each made major contributions to my thinking and continually amazed me in terms of what young human beings can accomplish when their minds are set free. The new generation free from Hillsdale College's PC conservatism—Dr. Robert Simpson, Todd Smith, Bill Kesterson, Michael Cornelius, Bill Killgallon, Tom Van Auken, Chris Cornelius, Mark Robinson, and Bret Talbot—are every bit as interesting to observe and much easier to teach as they find their piece of the path.

As to whether I have any writing skills, I'll allow the reader to make that judgment. I've a background in poetry which has allowed me to earn extra income as a designer of psychometric instruments and simulation games for heuristic purposes. My editors at North Atlantic Books, Kathy Glass and Sal Glynn, have been very helpful in correcting my failings and excesses. This is my first attempt at a complete work in easily readable prose. I have co-authored some textbooks, so my style leaves much to be desired. I am particularly indebted to Ms. Glass, who shows remarkable depth, humor, and insight.

Foreword

Dr. Morris and I met through the practice of Budo. Over the years, practicing together we have become close friends, which pleases me greatly. Dr. Morris has learned the Ninja way through observation and perceptive insight as he does not speak or read Japanese. He was able through his powers of empathy and observation to absorb and appreciate my natural behavior. In return, I have learned from observing his sharing way the application of American philosophy, psychology, and strategy.

No one can make conclusions about another's (or their own) actions. For example, logical actions may be effective, but there are times when drastic changes to the illogical add interest to one's life. Common sense is at times completely senseless.

What I have learned from Professor Morris's perspective is that the questing spirit (heart) when presented with illusory pathways will choose which path of many to take that leads to the one, and for this I am thankful. The behavior of the searcher or shugyo sha is one of total absorption and endurance. What follows is the devastation of one's own self, and in time the erasure of one's existence. This death is not the end but the start of the next spiritual phase—such as Jesus Christ showed in his resurrection.

The death of the socially learned self is the spiritual enlightenment or satori of Eastern beliefs. The business of the samurai is to die, but one reply of the samurai is to live on, renewed in nature. This is what I have gratefully learned from Dr. Morris.

The death that I speak of is a phase in our lives. This learning I have gained from my time with Busato Morris. By publishing this book he is explaining the importance of life as well as how to hold on to the energy of Life Force for human happiness and a natural, productive existence.

I hope that many people will read and gain from this book.
Masaaki Hatsumi, Bujin Tetsuzan: Soke, Bujinkan Ninpo
34th Grandmaster of Togakure Ryu Ninjutsu
Fourth year of Heisei, 9/30/92

Commentary

As usual I had three different translators work on Hatsumi's letter. I wanted to be certain I approximated his meanings as each translator's version was slightly different. I perceive Masaaki Hatsumi to be one of the great human beings in the world and his written and spoken words are to be studied carefully. All the translators complained about the difficulty of getting exact meaning from his use of archaic and tricky language. All agreed that what is above is close to the Japanese. I left in the Japanese term where I knew of no English equivalent or the translators varied widely in their interpretation. Once again I am indebted to Aikiko Tsao of Hillsdale College, Jeff Bristow of Jackson Community College and his living dictionary, an unnamed Japanese manager at CAMI products in Parma, Michigan.

Introduction to Enlightenment

In the summer of 1985 I began a series of experiments on myself following ancient Chinese and Japanese practices concerning the transformation of self. The result of this eclectic approach was the awakening of the kundalini, a very pronounced change in my perception, and a radical shift in physical health. Since the events of '85, I've developed a strong interest in Chinese traditional medicine and transpersonal psychology, as these two disciplines seemed to contain the most useful descriptions of what was/is happening to me as well as the best methods for protecting my sanity. I might add that very little of what I read at that time was particularly helpful, with the partial exception of Ken Wilber, John White, some tantric texts from Tibet, and Patanjali. The most useful information came from healers and martial artists. Only the martial artists seemed to exhibit the powers I was having to contend with and, depending on their degree of sophistication, had any understanding of the enormity of their gifts. As the years have gone by I have noted that many martial artists search for the esoteric in their art and find none. This book is meant to be a guide for them as to well as create some spirited discussion among the supposedly enlightened.

The *lesser kan and li* (opening the first four chakras or learning to run the microcosmic orbit) have become very easy to replicate in those who are willing to make the time to learn to breathe properly, and the transition to *Kundalini* is becoming so smooth that even the untrustworthy over-thirty crowd is going through it without taking damage. (Hindu term for connecting your genitals to your brain via the spinal column. The safer Chinese method for making this same energy connection is called the *greater kan and li*.) Just what implications the actualization of Western-educated enlightened masters holds is yet to be seen. Even the Chinese could not wish for more interesting times.

It is traditional for someone who is proposing a "way" to describe themselves or their lives so that followers may imitate them. I see little value in that exercise beyond establishing one's credentials, as my experiences leave me to believe that a teacher can only be a guide. If you're truly seeking enlightenment there comes a point when no master or scripture can help you, as you are on your own. However, as I work on this I will share whatever I feel is relevant but include my mistakes as well. Sometimes they're pretty funny but I expect you to make your own pratfalls. This is what *Musashi* (Japan's sword saint who wrote *The Book of Five Rings*) and others referred to when they declared they had no teachers.

You will have to find someone knowledgeable at some point to test your experience. I like banging heads with good martial artists. Adventure in the realm of *Sun Tzu* (ancient Chinese strategist who is credited with writing *The Art of War*) and the intuitive psyche through the purging fires of paranoia and other frightening and possibly liberating states of consciousness necessary to achieving flow in the martial arts isn't what most people are reaching for when they elect to put on canvas pajamas. Humanists, Transpersonal, and possibly Jungian therapists study the branches of psychology that are closest to dealing with the realities of the esoteric martial arts, which include disciplining the shadow when on the warrior path.

This book, following in the tradition started by *Lao Tzu* (purported author of *The Way of Power* or *Tao Te Ching*), is meant to be a guide for your thinking and practice. I will offer suggestions drawn from my own experience and that of my friends, and if they make sense to you—go for it. I will include nothing that I've not experienced myself. I will occasionally throw in a little code work for those who like to laugh with delight when they catch a riddle.

This book is structured according to the learning principles of the Hoshinroshiryu, which means some parts are written in the manner of a scroll. A scroll shows you the basic principles or formulas but expects you to complete the information in ways that work best for you. It is not a call for rote imitation. Each chapter is a layer of learning that helps you to understand the next chapter. The fundamentals are hardest and then by the time you're into the latter chapters you have the vocabulary and perspective to experiment with the meaning. I've attempted to illuminate the general theory and then follow the theory with applications or anecdotes that illustrate what has gone before. I am not going to footnote a lot of the research, but if you chase down the books offered in the bibliography you will be getting a graduate education in energy work and strategy. When you read a scroll without experiential knowledge of the subject matter, you will have difficulty unless you have an experienced teacher. One approaches a scroll from the viewpoint of a child—knowing nothing!

None of the chapters are truly meant to stand alone, but once you've read through the whole book, I highly recommend you try out some of the exercises with a good friend. You should not expect high-level results until you have mastered the meditation chapter and begun to develop your own source of internal chi. It is also my expectation that you become involved with a somatic art that will stretch you physically, as following the prescriptions in this text will move you mentally and spiritually. This is a grimmoire or cookbook for self-development. We begin by establishing credibility for the skeptical.

My Ph.D. is in Communication and my Sc.D. is in Psychology. I've worked most of my adult life as a teacher or consultant to Fortune 200 companies as a humanistic or third force (Maslow as opposed to Freud) psychologist. I've taught at major universities as well as a small private college and am once again teaching at a community college as well as accepting a dean's position with Eurotechnical Research University in Hilo, Hawaii, in The School of Polemikology. I've been married and divorced twice and raised six wannabe successful step-children. I've achieved master-level black belt rank in two esoteric martial arts (ninpo and chi kung) and earned black belt rank equivalents in combatic jujitsu and nei shen kung fu, as well as received honorary licenses in karate and kenpo. The lessons of aging, parenting, and marriage are similar but not equal to academic and martial ranks, as the standards for personal and social acceptance are somewhat higher than biological ability. I served as a medic in the U. S. Army during the Vietnam era but was fortunate enough to avoid the mass unit combat, spending most of my tour in Germany with the Third Infantry and then collecting my GI Bill. I've never been much of an athlete but was and am a compulsive reader. When I was a graduate teaching assistant at Penn State I was rated in the 98th percentile of all teachers at that university, somewhat to the chagrin of my advisers who thought I was shell-shocked.

I've always been a popular professor due not so much to grading policies, but to the originality of my viewpoint and dedication to sharing myself with my students. My teaching style is somewhat theatrical, as I've trained in theatre arts and believe a skilled teacher should be at least as interesting as television or why bother to have one. I strongly believe that education should be experientially structured where possible and that someone should only profess what they themselves have experienced. The experience does not have to be positive.

As I approach my fiftieth birthday I find myself with a seventh *dan* (black belt) ranking in *Bujinkan* (School of the Divine War Spirits) *Ninjutsu* (Intentional Skills) *Ninpo* (The Way of Intention) and the title of *Shidoshi* (master teaching license) , a sixth dan in Nihon karate jujitsu, and the title *Oshihan* (major master) granted by the *Bunbu I-Chi Zendo Budo Bugei Remmei* (the international organization for preserving the best scholarship concerning Japanese Zen traditions of conducting warfare or strategy), which is a bit embarrassing and difficult to live up to as a teacher of fundamentals. My eclectic skills of creating an actual working path to enlightenment (Hoshinroshiryu) have also been recognized by the *Dai Nippon Seibukan Remmei, Kokusai Budoin,* and the *Zen Kokusai Soke Budo Bugei Remmei* (Japanese organizations for traditional martial artists, of which I know little as ninjas are more secretive) and elected membership in The World Martial Arts Hall of Fame.

I'm delighted to be part of a new college specifically created for martial artists as dean of general academics for Eurotech's School of Polemikology.

Enlightenment is a biological process which has intellectual consequences. It can only be achieved through disciplining the body, which allows for the resurrecting of the spirit. Resurrecting the spirit means strengthening and entraining the body's electrochemical fields and hormonal systems normally thought of as the parasympathetic nervous systems and gaining control over the "flight/fight response." People familiar with esoteric or occult traditions may refer to this as opening and aligning the chakras, or if you've read into Taoist medical practice, running the micro- and macrocosmic orbits to "harmonize" the mind, spirit, and body. Religious people may experience this as union with god as the spirit gains ascendance. Yogis and ninjas both may refer to it as following the light, and Zen practitioners as following the breath.

I see enlightenment as a process of reeducating the mental structures which support the ego (the learned self and particularly the negative aspect sometimes referred to as the superego) to allow the id—which is grown up and housebroken though somewhat childish to run the show. The result is not psychosis but transcendence if the practitioner is altruistic, trusting, and *impeccable* (pursuing truth not perfection, not sinning, or missing the goal) in his or her practice of intention. Once the process starts it is almost impossible to stop, as it is a natural biological need to be righteous. Once startled out of "business as usual" the subconscious continuously seeks to awaken.

Behavior beyond the practice of meditation and integration has little to do with the path. If the practitioners are happy, relaxed, and confident they will follow their own path to enlightenment, which is also a peaceful heart. If not, they will follow others and this external focus may result in dependence, addiction, or paranoia depending on their chosen teacher. My basic position is we are not to worship but to become. Dr. Masaaki Hatsumi (thirty-fourth grandmaster of the Togakure Ryu) posits that the ninja's primary responsibility is spiritual development and a deep knowledge of all religions. I suggest a good course in cultural anthropology or comparative religion if you have only studied your own, or if you're sensible enough to have a secular or transcendent viewpoint, an examination of shamanistic practices across cultures may benefit your appreciation of some of the more esoteric aspects of ninpo.

As most of the techniques for spiritual development are drawn from religion it is necessary to understand that human beings and perhaps all living organisms are tripartite in that we all have mind, body, and spirit. Religion lays claim to responsibility for the spirit as science does for the mind and body. Religion is open to the same criticism as Skinnerian psychology. The socially learned self is shaped by the culture within which it is raised and thus only experiences the reality that is accepted for its group. In a modern industrial society consensus reality can be wildly complex, difficult to learn, and impossible to assimilate at all levels. Specialization and mastery are rewarded as they are replicable. Generalization, abstraction, and intuition are recognized by the wise, but as they are seen so rarely, may or may not be rewarded.

Intuition is often seen as female or left handed. In some cultures, even today, left-handed children are allowed to die at birth ensuring a more manageable left-brained population, which is more amenable to extrinsic logic. Whereas the left-handed raised in a right-handed world have to be more creative, ambidextrous, and use more of their brains in order to survive. The left is considered female and clumsy in a right-handed world. Creativity is seldom rewarded in traditional martial arts, which often slavishly follow the example of their founder. The traditional ways are nearly all right-handed. Tantrism is sometimes referred to as the left-handed way, as it forces one to transgress accepted social beliefs to deepen one's experience of reality. Some aspects of ninjutsu are influenced by tantrism.

In Western society higher IQs are associated with left-handedness and myopia from reading. Leonardo Da Vinci, Michelangelo, and Picasso were lefties, as are many professional athletes, particularly in baseball. Spiritual death of the learned self is supposed to come from the left. Death of the ego is necessary to true enlightenment. The death of the ego or male right frees the intuition or the female left. Every enlightened martial artist that I've met has been left- handed or ambidextrous. Androgyny and ambidexterity as well as gentility are related. Learning to use both sides of your body opens areas of brain function, as it stimulates the nervous system. As we learn best that which gives us pleasure, it is important to choose a form of exercise which is perceived as pleasurable fun for you. Natural, relaxed, efficient body movement is essential to enlightenment as well as to developing the "chi" or "ki" or "wa" or "spirit"(different names for living energy) necessary for the *siddhis* (eight natural psychic abilities) or magic. Flexibility is also critical as "sound mind—sound body" can be jumped to "flexible body—flexible mind."

Physical flexibility is required to avoid injury in the martial arts and is emphasized in the more difficult softer arts such as tai chi or taijutsu or yoga. These are particularly beneficial for preparing the body for the changes that will occur as the process of enlightenment progresses. Rejuvenation of the endocrine system results in change.

If you are right-handed, start doing things left-handed. If you are a dedicated left-hander, start using your right. At every opportunity stretch and maneuver your spine and neck. Most of us don't seem to realize our brain is part of our spine and as Voltaire said, "only what we think we think with." The brain is part of the central nervous system. It extends from the top of our heads to the tip of our tails with less gross extensions to all extremities of our bodies. In other words no mind/body dichotomy. Stretching, dance, yoga, and *shiatsu* (massage techniques that affect the body's bioelectrical systems) can all be important tools for disciplining the body in a relaxed, pleasurable way.

An important point many seekers miss is that the more relaxed you are, the more efficiently the spirit can move within the body. Physical strength is nice but at a certain point muscularity gets in the way of self -development. You may notice that none of the *godan* and above in ninjutsu have the physical presence of an Arnold Schwarzenegger or Jean-Claude Van Damme (famous actors). If you are going to be a spy or gatherer of intelligence, an outstanding build is too easily identified.

Internal exercises drawn from Chinese medicine to develop healing energy are becoming better known in the West. Esoteric yogas that teach the practitioner how to use the sacrum and skull as pumps, the intestines as storage coils, and the blood, bones, and meridians as conduits are more effective for developing real power than lifting weights and have the additional benefit of activating the hormonal systems, which greatly slows the aging process, hence the more reasonable claims for longevity or immortality. This rejuvenation is best accomplished through active control of the breath. I've noticed that since going through the kundalini I only take about four breaths a minute.

In the course of this book I will have to discuss religion, psychology, meditation, physical practice, psychic phenomena, channeling, teaching and learning theory and relate those to the martial arts in general and to the study of ninpo in particular. People tell me my viewpoint is not shared by many. There will be times when what I discuss will contradict traditional practice, and some of what I talk about can only be understood through experience. I strongly recommend trying out the exercises from an attitude of no expectations and then carefully monitor your progress with a diary.

May I also state very clearly my goal was never to become a ninja but to advance myself as a human being. Ninjutsu is one of my hobbies, what I measure myself and my students against, and it is probably the only surviving combat-oriented Mystery School whose traditions have not been warped or lost because it's still operating and transforming the dangerous into the beautiful. Masaaki Hatsumi is a living buddha, gentleman, scholar, artist, doctor, actor, enduring fighter, good friend, and a lot of fun. This book is not about how to become a ninja, or a martial artist, but it is about mastery of subtle differences, inner adventuring, and what that might mean for you as a human animal attempting to become a complete human being by transcending your culture and your animal self. Stephen Hayes asked me one time as we were riding around in Japan what I thought of ninjutsu. My reply was, "Ninjutsu is the most effective way of dealing with violent paranoids that I've ever seen."

Learning ninjutsu has given me the opportunity to observe what happens when other Westerners get sucked into real spiritual training. Hatsumi-san is a living Buddha. The names of the nine living traditions that are subsumed by ninpo and manifested in his expression of Bujinkan Ninpo have names associated with Eastern sorcery and mysticism. As the names of the schools *(ryus)* suggest, these are not trivial subjects and there are parallels in Western mysticism. A knowledge of esoteric terminology from traditional Chinese medicine might give you an indication that if you are going to study in this graduate school . . . hang on to your hat, as the ride is going to get pretty interesting! (More about these schools in the next chapter.) Many American ninjas have only learned the Japanese sounds in naming these schools without researching their meaning, as if pronunciation were more important than understanding. They're the most fun to watch over time as their terror becomes visible to the compassionate view of those who have gone before them.

Ninpo is the equivalent of a graduate school for the person who can only negotiate nonverbally with a terrorist. We forget that historically the ninja warrior from the Togakure Ryu was regarded as a sorcerer, and folklore associates them with ruling over the *tengu* (demonic, raven-like spirits haunting the mountains in Japan). There is a very real shamanistic core to Bujinkan Ninpo that transcends ninjutsu.

Chapter One

A Brief History of Ninjutsu, Ancient and Modern

TOGAKURE RYU NINJUTSU was founded by Daisuke Togakure after winding up on the losing side of a revolt against the oppressive Heike regime in Japan some 800 years ago. Daisuke Togakure was a noble with responsibilities to his people. He could be considered a country samurai. He barely escaped with his life. In Japan, the losers in a war against the state are supposed to commit *seppuku* (ritual suicide). He didn't do that. He ran like a woman back up the mountain into the forests to warn and hide his children. He took what he learned from the awful experience of watching most of his friends hunted down and slashed to pieces and began a school that teaches how to survive against overwhelming odds when every hand is turned against you and those in positions of authority consider you to be cowardly, of the wrong religion, and an impostor. The Japanese treat history with a revisionist eye now and did in the past, too. The ninja *ryus* remained underground for nearly a thousand years.

Hiding in the sewers can lead to associations with the rat, spider, and night moves. In that time much knowledge was gained and lost. The Koga ryus, which emphasized combatic training only, had no spiritual component beyond Zen but were able to create many interesting systems of defense and penetration and estab-

1

lished a reputation for teamwork and assassination. To the best of my knowledge no Koga school still exists as an unbroken ryu, but there are teachers who can share bits and pieces of their ancient lore. I am told that members of the Koga ryus consider Masaaki Hatsumi a traitor for teaching gaijin and revealing the secret training. This could be compared to Bruce Lee's revealing wu shu to Westerners, but the order of revelation is cosmic in comparison.

The Togakure Ryu—according to my informant Hanshi Richard Kim, something of a martial arts historian—broke away from the Koga ryus to establish a school for enlightened warriors who operated as individuals practicing Ninpo (suffix designating a combat-proven way to enlightenment with Chinese roots) over ninjutsu. Takamatsu, the thirty-third grandmaster, was a spy in China for the Japanese during World War II. He was president of the Japanese *Busen* (professional scholars of the arts of war) in China and studied and demoed with many fine Chinese martial artists during the years of Japan's brutal occupation. There are many harrowing tales concerning his valor. Like many ancient samurai, when confronted with the darker side of their quest he, too, became a Shingon Buddhist priest in his later years. He was a family man and provided a good life for his spouse and daughter. Takamatsu's paintings reveal a childlike sense of humor, and Hatsumi-*san* (suffix denoting respectful friendship) describes him as a fiercely tender teacher.

The first task of the Togakure Ryu ninja is spiritual refinement by whatever means necessary. For some facing their mirror is a fearful nightmare. For others it is the *Musubi* (knot similar to the Gordion that Alexander the Great cut with his mother's sword). It is to be examined layer by layer, for it holds great treasures. It is imaginatively similar in shape to the brain, but leaving the tail hanging would give too great a clue to its nature for a riddle for the not-too-bright, but gutsy. Interpreting legends often provides interesting insights into our own lives, as evidenced by Joseph Campbell's popularity among the spiritually misled.

Masaaki Hatsumi began sharing his expression of the complete art of ninpo in the early seventies and has shared a body of knowledge in Bujinkan that is unmatched in my experience (I have been involved with martial arts for thirty-seven years). Many people regard ninjutsu with great suspicion, primarily because they have been exposed to the viewpoint of the competition, or had the sour experience of being taught by a psychopathic fraud. Ninpo is a living art with an awe-inspiring reputation as a route to enlightenment as well as a system of self-protection par excellence. As I was given a Shidoshi's license by Hatsumi-*soke* (suffix meaning grandmaster), passed the sword test for fifth dan in 1990, and was granted a *nanaedan* or *shichidan's* license (seventh) in 1992, you can take my commentary with some degree of credibility.

There are other practitioners who have far greater taijutsu skills than I and some who have studied years longer. But as a Ph.D. and a psychologist focusing on the transpersonal who has been through the greater kan and li or kundalini, my perspective may be more objective than most, as I only consider ninjutsu my hobby and Hatsumi-*sensei* (suffix indicating a teacher/student relationship) my rather odd friend. As I do not take friendship lightly I feel no guilt at turning my concentration toward him, as he has shared much with his American students in a very honest and open manner. He is very approachable but really expects you to learn his language. He butchers English far better than I can even contemplate mangling Japanese. I think he spends a lot of time on his riddles and koans. He does some things that make you think hard for a long time.

Ninjas are emotional people with deep attachments. His American organization is growing through the skill of the Bujinkan teachers, and the screening of the guard is becoming harder to penetrate. Ninpo is far more challenging and interesting than golf, bowling, tennis, or Vipassana meditation. It took me five years to get from white belt to ninth kyu green belt—I already had considerable experience in karate, jujitsu, kung fu, and Zen meditation and was beginning to learn Tao Tien Chi Kung. I still consider myself a beginner in ninpo after ten years. It is difficult to give up wrong practice when you learned it young. However, the tools I have taken from ninjutsu have bolstered my strengths and provided time and distance for my weaknesses.

Taijutsu is the physical art associated with ninpo. Because its roots are Chinese, real ninjutsu looks a great deal like the softer Chinese martial arts performed with a more Japanese linear body movement necessary to wearing armor. After thousands of years, the art of taijutsu is, of course, thought of as Japanese. The low stances and lunging body movements of the beginner are modified with time and experience into much more subtle and hard-to-see movements so that the seasoned veteran has exquisite balance and power but in no way resembles a fighter. (Taking deep stances and yelling "kiai" when you are in enemy territory is hardly a sign of skilled intelligence.) You can see this by contrasting the videos of Bussey's Warrior International with any of Hatsumi's Quest videos or the videos available from Greg Kowalski of actual ninja training in Japan by Hatsumi-soke and his *Shihan* (master teachers who have experienced the lesser kan and li). Once you have witnessed real Bujinkan Ninjutsu you are usually deeply impressed by its flow and how much it does *not* look like Tae kwan do, Okinawan karate as typically taught, aikido, or jujitsu but does look like some of the combatic kung fu.

The flow of the art is unique and subtle. I might also add that many of the moves are surprisingly funny and take advantage of the more rigid styles' favorite attacks and ways of wearing armor and weapons. The ninjas' traditional enemy was an arrogant, over-bearing, well-fed and exercised, armor-clad, sword-bearing samurai who was a product of one of the kenjutsu ryus. Techniques that failed the test of actual application were not passed on, for torture, interrogation, and death greeted the inept, as the Togakure Ryu intelligence gatherer worked alone under the sword of his opponent. The gatherer of intelligence must serve at least two masters well or his or her information will be tainted.

The *katas* (memorized forms) or *Kihon Hoppo* (basic moves) in ninjutsu are quite short by Chinese standards (usually five moves) but can be adapted to the eight directions and various weapons in every case. Each of the nine ryus that Masaaki Hatsumi has brought under the umbrella of Togakure Ryu Bujinkan Ninpo has its own Kihon Hoppo variations which can keep the enthusiast busy and happy for a very long time. There are some slight differences from teacher to teacher as to what is considered a base of knowledge worthy of reaching the next *kyu* or *dan* rank. The fundamentals vary from year to year as your experience grows and in relation to what point in the teaching cycle you entered the system. The Israeli ranking system used throughout Canada is slightly different from the Kasumi-An ranks used by Stephen Hayes's Nine Gates or Shadows of Iga methods. Detroit Bujinkan—where I play most often—draws its ranking system from tenth dan Daron Navon (Israeli) as well as Greg Kowalski (seventh dan) and Larry Turner (sixth dan) and is supervised by Shidoshi-ho Otto Cardew, a very knowledgeable sandan (third-degree black belt).

With few exceptions ninjas wear traditional black *dogi* (canvas pajamas) and *tabi* (spit-toed, cloth boots with a thin, corrugated, flexible sole) while training. The hooded night suits popularized by the theatre and media are usually not worn. Those are actually the suits worn by prop managers in Japanese theatre productions which convention renders invisible when they walk onstage to move a prop. The belt system for adults consists of white, nine *kyus* (pre-black belt ranks) of green, and ten *dans* (degrees) of black. Fifth-degree black belt and above (master level rank and a special certification for teaching, *shidoshi*) can *only* be awarded by the Grandmaster Masaaki Hatsumi in Bujinkan, Togakure Ryu Ninjutsu. Grades of black belt are distinguished by the chest patch, not belt stripes or color change. A master's patch is red, with the kanji and perimeter surrounded by a white border. A shihan's patch includes yellow and green to represent the opening of the heart and solar plexus chakras.

All dan ranking diplomas in Bujinkan are hand-brushed in Japanese and have red seals stamped on them identifying Hatsumi as well as the particular ryus. The cover of this book is from my godan license. As there are less than a hundred Americans who have attained master ranking in Bujinkan Ninpo at this time, most of the thousands of people who purport to teach traditional ninjutsu are frauds of various stripe. You may take this book along when you go shopping for a teacher.

Tannemura, who actually claims to be Takamatsu's successor, is an interesting break-away from Hatsumi who was never able to understand the spiritual side of ninpo. He claims to be the true grandmaster of the Togakure Ryu but is given no credence in Japan. I have seen the scrolls of Takamatsu at the shidoshi training in Japan and had Japanese friends read them to me while Hatsumi looked on. A master passes his scroll to his successor so that his exact thoughts will be preserved; there is also the transfer of spirit at death to be considered, and I have seen the spirit of Takamatsu-sensei in company with Hatsumi-soke. Time is of little importance when expressing genius. Physical skill does not always correspond to mental and seldom to spiritual.

At the end of this chapter I'll praise some teachers I admire, and you can follow up as you like. The real thing is worth pursuing, and even a hobbyist can have a great time studying ninjutsu. The Warrior International Network (P.O. Box 30338, Stockton, CA 95213) has recently published a directory for $5 of quite a few legitimate teachers and enthusiasts listed by state. This is a big country and the good teachers are thin on the ground. Spellers, too, as you will see when you get to my entry.

Ninpo is a living art and that means the shidoshi-level teachers are all artists of a very physical nature with their own creative viewpoint being exercised to bring the traditional learnings of the schools into alignment with their own personality and the reality of our times. This means that dogi are sometimes replaced with cammies when people are training in the woods or street clothes when training in town. I have even seen the clever application of camouflage to wetsuits for UDT work. I have seen people do some very risky and stupid things thinking they were getting real ninja training because weapons and cammies were involved. The ninja usually trains outside a great deal of time under clement and inclement weather conditions. Some of the most fun I've had has been training with Shihan Kevin Millis (seventh dan) on the beaches below Malibu as well as working on climbing techniques in Joshua Tree. One learns the traditional weapons and tools and then their modern adaptations and applications. It's fun to know

6

how to shoot a flintlock or even make one, but my military experience has taught me considerable respect for communication, aviation, artillery, armor, and automatic weapons. Being invisible when the heavy-weapon folks are around is very useful. Sun Tzu has some very interesting philosophical positions that are well understood and brought to life in the practice of ninpo.

Training in a combat-oriented martial art is a gift that is meant to save your life. It can be regarded as a means for taking the lives of others but that is a perversion of the Way. Some people can only see it in that perspective. I would not like to live in their bodies nor share their poor blighted spirits. To quote Patton, "The object of this battle is to let the other poor dumb son of a bitch die for his country." A martial artist wants to live, not die gloriously. Patton wouldn't even let his troops dig foxholes, as he considered them little graves. Movement was his forté. He taught the Nazis blitzkrieg as a total concept; their racist stupidity would never see a Red Ball Express run by a subject race. Training in an art designated as a "jutsu" indicates the focus is on combat techniques not sport. The knowledge passed on is to keep you alive and well when others are attempting to kill you. Arts that have a "po" suffix have ancient roots in China and usually a concealed developmental component as well as combatic techniques. Arts designated as "do" are supposed to be concerned with developing the self as well as providing a path to enlightenment. I cannot think of any "do" which has not been perverted by sport in the United States and know of no master living today who achieved full enlightenment following the precepts of that suffix. You have to observe closely.

A teacher provides the skills from his or her experience. The student learns to apply the lessons from their viewpoint. A poor teacher can only convey technique. A great teacher inspires desire to learn with feelings, technique, and self-discovery. A learner soon recognizes fear and hatred are a waste of time and spirit. Only lovers achieve completeness. Love is a learned behavior that is biologically motivated. It's easy to learn when you love what you're doing. Commitment is not the same, but bears a close relationship. One is often preparation for the other. Teaching is often erotic in nature when the student and teacher are deeply involved in the subject matter. This is seldom discussed but certainly is true. It is the major reason why so many professors marry their graduate students or have affairs with them.

The traditional skills and eighteen levels of training for a ninja are listed in Hatsumi's *Ninjutsu: History and Tradition* (Unique Publications, 1981). Masaaki Hatsumi, Stephen Hayes, and Jack Hoban have published a whole series of excellent books on ninjutsu with Contemporary Books. Hayes also published a good series of five basic readers with Ohara that are collector's items now but have just been reissued with gorgeous covers by Greg Manchess. A careful examination of these works does not reveal the unemotional, heartless assassin so often associated with ninjutsu in the popular media by Ashida Kim, Frank Ducs, and Eric von Lustbader, but an extremely well thought out defense system stretching from the individual to the community, having medical, intellectual, political, geographical, and social aspects of survival taken into consideration, particularly from the underdog's viewpoint. The ninja spent a lot more time figuring out how to get out of the ropes than how to tie someone up. (Now that I think about it, I've only had classes in escaping in ninjutsu. You were allowed to tie your own knots.) Kirtland C. Peterson's *Mind of the Ninja* (Contemporary Books, 1986) gives an excellent analysis of the *omote* (exterior) concepts and behavioral patterns of the ninja as presented in modern society from a Western and Jungian perspective.

Stephen Turnbull's recent book on ninjutsu completely glosses over the fact that many of the old prints shown there refer to the men and women identified as ninjas as royalty. His text goes on to identify them as Chinese bandits and outlaws who followed Sun Tzu. An extremely secondary-source viewpoint. It's like having a lowbrow Japanese tell you what Koreans are like, or a Klansman describe Jews, or a practitioner of a sport-based martial art with lots of rules give you an opinion of a combat-based art with no rules. My father, who was a collegiate champion boxer and wrestler, still contemptuously refers to my interests as "Oriental Dirty Fighting." This is after nearly forty years, senility excused, and what he thinks of as judo.

The classical ninja according to Hatsumi—and I have no reason to doubt him as I've had some very interesting experiences hanging out with the upper level ninji—was a mystic, and the Japanese version is not very different from our Western version. The Togakure ninja worked at developing a deep and accurate self-knowledge, and from that mystical perspective of universality granted by satori only engaged in combat when motivated by discovery, love, or reverence. (Righteous warriors are to be greatly feared, as we well know in the West, seeking always to have God on our side.) Spiritual refinement was the primary skill for the traditional ninja of the Togakure Ryu. Taijutsu or unarmed combat skills involving striking, kicking, avoiding, blocking, grappling, choking, and escaping the holds of others as well as leaping, rolling, silent movement, and tumbling were secondary skills. Tertiary knowledge of the sword and a whole slew of other skills, like weapons and pharmacopoeia, continue the list. Like the Okinawans, there were periods when the mountain people were not allowed weapons or at least swords by their rulers. The ninja treat weapons as tools for the most part, and the use and creation of unorthodox and concealed weaponry is part of the training.

There's always some debate as to who are teachers of legitimate ninjutsu. If your instructor is putting more emphasis on teaching you how to capture somebody rather than how to get away, I would suggest the lessons of warfare against the government have not yet sunk in. Of course you have to know the former to really accomplish the latter. If all he can do is tie them up then your education is incomplete should you be captured or hunted. Escaping is critical if you screwed up enough to be attacked or got aggressive yourself. I throw that in for the handcuffs and feathers crowd.

The old kanji in the names of the nine ryus have esoteric meanings which were translated for me by Mark Lithgow, an Englishman and translator who lives in Noda City, Japan. He has been a student of ninpo for many years and works often with Masaaki Hatsumi as a translator. The esoteric titles are: The School of the Hidden Door (or Mysterious Portal) ; School of the Jeweled Tiger; The Immovable School Passed Down from the Gods; The Enlightening School Wrested from the Nine Demon Gods; Tiger Felling Dragon School; The School of the Hidden Cloud; The School of the Jeweled Heart; Water and Mountain Spirit Rules; and The Takagi Tree Felling School. Bujinkan can be translated as "The School of the Divine Warriors," as well as "War Spirit Building." Shidoshi can be translated as "Knight of the Four Ways," or "Teacher of the Ways of Life and Death." (As you may guess from the names, this is not the equivalent of a Harvard MBA even for a Japanese.) My translation of Mark's translation goes this way:

The Way of the Hidden Door. You have to go through the door that is concealed to learn anything. That which conceals the door is something we don't want to look at. In Taoism the corresponding school is called Mysterious Portal, and one of its meanings is to use your rectum as an energy pump when you're moving sexual energy up your spine. The Hindu correspondent has to do with using *chitta* (living energy which can be directed by the mind) to hide yourself or build an energy tunnel toward your goal with the *ajna* (third eye/forehead chakra). The third eye is considered a doorway to enlightenment. You can't see it until you have it. Sometimes as it opens one experiences an interesting form of tunnel vision that is like looking into a doorway into another dimension, which it may be.

The Way of the Jeweled Tiger. Tiger refers to goddess or yin energy, which flows up the front of the body. When a person knows how to see energy, the acupuncture or shiatsu points glow, as well as the chakras, on a harmonized, powerful person and look like little Christmas tree lights or jewels as the energy flows through, sometimes also creating a striped effect along the meridians. There is a method for striping your aura that works as camouflage at night.

The Immovable School Passed Down from the Gods. This has to do with the stilling of the mind. Once you have "killed your ego" you have total control of your emotional states. You cannot be swayed from your purposes. The preferred state is neutrality or no desires—*mushin* or no-mind. The "way of death" is a little sexual joke in both the samurai and ninja traditions and actually refers to subduing the personality or learned self. Once you've accomplished this you are considered a living buddha and able to draw inspiration from those fierce enlightened ones who have gone before you. In the West you might be considered a god of rock and roll (Clapton).

The Water or Mountain Rules or Spirit Building School. Water is another term for living energy, and the student of this school seems to flow like water, as does the sexual energy and blood. One of the monster dragons in Chinese lore has a bowl of water balanced on its head. *Kappa* (sprite/animal spirits that appear almost human) in Japanese fairy tales were water gnomes who had the power to knit bones and regrow tissue. Water is a code word for chi, or in Japanese *ki,* or spirit. The name suggests flow or movement with power. Rules imply danger. It might also be translated as Mountain Water. That analogy should be powerful and clear. Mountain is a code term for yang sexual energy.

The Enlightening School Wrested from the Nine Demon Gods. I love this name. It's rather like the seven deadly sins plus two. Energy has to move up to the brain for enlightenment to take place, and an enlightened being should rule his or her own demons as well as have understanding and compassion for the foibles of others. I would expect an emphasis on opening the chakras as well as controlling the emotions, with a rich smattering of Machiavellian-like psychology. This school name reflects a yin or darker curriculum. The ninja must understand both the positive and negative aspects of power, where the so-called saint tries to ignore the darker aspects of being human and sees martyrdom as a worthy goal. Inner deities or chakras are sometimes considered demons. Living energy can appear demonic or angelic. A demon god is someone who rules demons.

Tiger Felling Dragon School. Yang energy or dragon energy is considered male. This is an exercise in male chauvinism. Yin is

11

considered female since it is attractive, whereas yang is repelling. This school focuses on the subconscious subsuming the ego or learned self. Learning to be soft and supple like a female. Learning how to receive an attack and turn it to your own use. Learning to use your left side. On another level it may mean the absorption of the sperm's energy for chi, resulting in the death of sexual desire or the little swimmers' ability to go very far. This can be considered too effective a means of birth control if you're interested in having children. You might want to wait a while before studying in this school. Conversely, some of the tantric techniques are reputed to re-energize the sperm. Consult Mantak Chia's books and/or Douglas and Slinger's *Sexual Secrets* (Aurora). Hatsumi's war name of White Dragon connotes androgyny. There is a school of kung fu named White Tiger Swallows Green Dragon, as well as a very nasty women's school called Black Tiger.

The School of the Hidden Cloud. In the material world this could be thought of as all the ninja's nifty blinders and powders, as well as trickery and deceit to cloud the mind of an opponent. Because the aura looks like a cloud around the individual, I suspect this is where that knowledge finds its home.

The Way of the Jeweled Heart. Opening of the heart chakra is second only to the kundalini in the achievement of enlightenment. In the West we say "follow your heart" when we advise others to do their best in difficult situations. It is associated with wind techniques in the Go Dai and the personality trait of benevolence or open acceptance. In Taoist esoteric yoga the heart is connected to the tongue. When your heart is open it is very difficult to lie. Many wind techniques are specifically for receiving your opponent's attack openly with benevolence so you can take a prisoner or restrain a friend.

The Takagi Tree Felling School. Probably the most forthright in terminology unless I've missed something. Trees are blown down by the wind. Chi again. As one of my early senseis used to try to tell me, "When the big wind comes, the mighty oak falls but the willow bends with the breeze." I was eighteen and in the army. My kindest thought was that Orientals are eccentric. Full-body taijutsu uprooting movement probably comes out of here. In Kurosawa's *The Seven Samurai,* one of the seven makes a joke about this legendary school.

I once had a long talk with a Japanese sociologist who was amazed that I was studying real ninjutsu. When she looked at the *kanji* (Japanese iconographs) on the diploma she said they were very, very old, of a type not used in Japan for centuries. She also said that Iga Province was where all the wild people were sent as punishment during the Warring States Period. Since its mountains are now a well-preserved ski area, the wild people are still enjoying frightening the samurai flatlanders.

As a means of disguising from the enemy the real purpose of these schools, under the discipline of *kyojitsu* (telling lies that appear to be the truth), each mental and spiritual practice was hidden within a physical or weapon technique. You can master the physical techniques of ninjutsu without having a clue to the mental disciplines. You can also learn the mental disciplines without being shown the internal energy uses. You can't learn ninpo without taijutsu, however.

For example, each of the *kamae* or fighting postures, which are normally treated as end products of exemplary movement when applying a technique or avoiding one, are also *asanas* or yogic postures that if held and used for meditation greatly strengthen the body and develop one's sense of balance far beyond normal limits. The physical postures strengthen the spine and encourage the body's electrical systems, while the rolling techniques add to one's flexibility and mobility. When the physical posture is enlivened by an attitude appropriate to that way of standing or being we refer to it as *flow* or *integration,* which is often the compelling effect of being completely natural. When done properly, ninjutsu is totally based on natural, relaxed body movement flowing from the subconscious mind without intellectual intervention. In that, it is closely related to tai chi or nei shen kung Fu.

The use of the breath and energy is not discussed in ninjutsu in my experience with the Japanese beyond a simple discussion of different *kiai.* That knowledge is only passed from grandmaster to grandmaster. You may have noted reading Musashi that when he really wants you to get studying he uses the disclaimer of "oral tradition." However, any chi kung practitioner who has advanced to the macrocosmic orbit will find taijutsu an excellent medium for moving energy.

In the six years I've been observing him Hatsumi has only slipped once and mentioned chi. He was showing a technique for unbalancing someone wearing armor at the Atlanta Tai Kai in 1990 when he said "To make this work you must move your chi down to your feet." It sent his *uke* (training partner who receives and hopes to survive a training experience) sailing. The statement was edited out of the video. Don't expect a ninja to teach you chi kung. You are supposed to figure that part of the formula out yourself by going into yourself. I asked Daron Navon (tenth dan) about teaching some of this at a seminar, and he said it was too difficult. When I told Hatsumi I couldn't honestly teach ninjutsu without teaching chi kung he replied by giving me a shidoshi license. (In my opinion it is the only Way and I personally recommend the Chinese National Chi Kung Institute.) They had to censor the hell out of this year's Tai Kai video, as Hatsumi-sensei gave away secrets that most of us who were privileged to see will have to work years to get down smoothly. I usually settle for the pragmatic and have been accused of sacrificing green belts to increase my knowledge of how to give pain. I'm a hobbyist and like the short path.

The field of battle is outside the dojo. Only four people that I know of have been killed outside the dojo in training accidents, and I know of no one being permanently maimed or crippled by a master instructor. You are not paying fees to be injured unless that is the only way you will learn. There are many people who put on fatigues or night suits and claim to teach authentic ninjutsu. I was told by one fraud in Toledo, Ohio, that Steve Hayes had given him his red sash in Yin/Yang ninjutsu (my pregnant ass). Only Hatsumi gives the sword test, and there are no red sashes in Togakure Ryu ninjutsu. Nor were there any Kasumi-An diplomas or Bujinkan licenses in his dojo, just a lot of students being ripped off. I occasionally run into a young ninjutsu trainee in Chicago bringing bad and acting macho with his *tabi* (funny feet for scufflers) when I'm out partying. It's pretty obvious he has missed the concept of humility and doesn't understand the true value and danger of invisibility. He brags about his taijutsu and attempts to frighten people. Eventually someone will shoot him. Most Togakure Ryu dojo attempt to follow the tradition of providing some guidance in etiquette, but many students in the U.S.A. have little exposure to the practice of dangerous adult human beings treating each other with respect.

Kevin Millis, who teaches out of Irvine, California, is a great teacher and I recommend him highly for those who live on the west coast. In the Northeast, Greg Kowalski in Wallingford, Connecticut, has taught me many things and I treasure his friendship. Mark Davis in Boston runs a good school. The best bang for your buck in the Midwest can be found near Ann Arbor. Shidoshi-ho Otto Cardew supervises the U of M's as well as Schoolcraft College's ninjutsu clubs and gives private lessons at his home dojo. I've enjoyed Otto's rough-and-ready brand of taijutsu training for over ten years. Larry Turner, out of Dayton Ohio, conducts excellent seminars. Tucker, Georgia, a suburb of Atlanta, hosts Bud Malmstrom, the highest-ranked American ninja, who has excellent teaching skills and even a large children's contingent. Stephen Hayes still teaches out of Germantown, Ohio. There are some very good technicians in Texas, but I've never attended any of their trainings, just seen them perform at Tai Kais.

If you are planning an adventure of going to Japan to train, I would recommend traveling with Millis or Kowalski. If you want to soak up the historical culture and see the sights, Stephen Hayes leads some interesting tours. Toshiro Nogato teaches in Tokyo. Tetsuji Ishizuka is in Kashiwa City and both speak English. I sent my son-in-law to train with Ishizuka when he was stationed near Tokyo with the U.S. Marines. You really should have an invitation or escort before you impose yourself on Shiraishi-sensei or Masaaki Hatsumi-soke in Noda City. I've seen visiting martial artists show up uninvited in Noda and expect to be provided for as if they were visiting V.I.P.s. Only ninja kindness kept them from suffering for their foolishness. In the next chapter I discuss chi kung from a martial arts perspective and relate that to the kundalini.

Chapter Two

Chi Kung and Kundalini: The Real Secret of The Masters

WORTHWHILE MARTIAL ARTS have a basis in meditation and chi kung. Usually the secrets of chi are not passed down until the student has spent long years proving his or her worthiness of the gift. There are many techniques for transmission and generation of chi but all require a master-student relationship unless you are inclined to intense self-study. Self-study is the source of unique gifts and often requires conquering your greatest fears. According to Sun Tzu, self-adventure also results in the greatest powers. Only time will tell, but there are probably more accomplished people doing esoteric studies on their own right now than at any time in human history. Mantak Chia's many books on Taoist esoteric practice provide excellent information on this little-understood area in the higher-level martial arts that is the equivalent of the kundalini in yoga.

I was rereading Gopi Krishna's description of his kundalini experience and also listening to Christina Grof's tape on her experiences (by Sounds True). In both cases we have adventurers experiencing an internal journey for which neither has a map. Gopi Krishna takes almost twenty years to "kill his ego" and get on with absorption into the void but was severely handicapped by having to rely on ancient scriptures and coded directions left by long-dead masters who had probably passed on the warnings orally. He was also handicapped by having to work alone, as all of the great spiritual leaders of his generation had not fulfilled their task of achieving enlightenment. Nobody knew what to do. The Jungian analysis that accompanies his text is occasionally helpful, but also completely misses the point considering Gopi Krishna's call to experimentation and *replication* (scientific term for repeating the experiment with similar results).

The methods for bringing to fruition the kundalini, like many techniques in the martial arts, are easily learned if seen or shown but would never be done if the neophyte didn't happen on the right combination by accident. Gopi Krishna describes the terror of the body's natural energy arising and the effects that it had on him because of his minimal preparation. Most people reading the book are not drawn to experiencing the light when made aware of the fact that you can shine or burn.

The opening to energy and being able to move your center out into the fields often results in experiences that could be considered "psychic," such as sharing another person's perceptions, thoughts, and feelings. As each chakra is opened by the sexual energy moving up the spine, a different perspective (personality) is formed of the world out of the emergent feelings. Continuing the climb through conscious direction has often been analogized to mountain climbing, with the movement into the energy realms as ascent into heaven. If nothing else it provides ample proof to the adventurers that there is an aspect of themselves that has little to do with the body.

Mr. Krishna makes it quite clear the experience nearly killed him on a number of occasions but for the ministrations of his wife. He didn't have a clue as to how to prepare his body for higher energy beyond pushing the energy from the genitals up the spine. Ms. Grof's adventures are received with better humor as she has been at least exposed to a *saddhu* who is not a benevolent fraud and has a notion that if she doesn't go insane there is a worthwhile goal or light somewhere up ahead. It also helped to have the support of her husband, a rather famous researcher in transpersonal psychology and LSD, who has modernized some of the ancient techniques for transcendence into what he refers to as "holographic breath training." Their Spiritual Emergence Network provides a very real service for those who are battling their inner demons.

I mention these two as well known examples of contemporary people who have experienced the inner awakening without benefit of martial arts training. This can happen to anyone who meditates in an upright position regardless of gender if they're beyond puberty. In the martial arts the training of the breath energy is referred to as chi kung and the awakening of the kundalini as the *greater kan and li* (Chinese) or *entering the void* (Japanese). Transmission of the secrets of generation was usually from father to son, mother to daughter in family systems, or to a chosen disciple when bloodlines were not essential as in the Togakure Ryu. The secrets of generation and transmission were closely held, as the benefits of success—greater creativity, endurance, longevity, compassion and psychic advantages—greatly benefited the family or training group. The person who can best absorb the grandmaster's energy and accept the Bujin without going crazy is considered a lineage heir. In Bujinkan Ninpo the role of grandmaster skips a generation so the successor has time to learn his or her role and be trained by the best of the previous generation.

As spiritual development and the generation of healing internal energy are usually regarded as the property of the religions and viewed as the heroic and never mythological characteristics of the saints and founders, not ordinary people—a little secrecy was probably in order. In the West we had the human alchemists and Masonic lodges. In modern times, Taliesen as founded by the Wrights and adherence to the Gurdjieff model would parallel the *ryus* and *kwoons* of Asia as training halls for the artistic spirit, or warrior heart. I consider the *Hoshinroshiryu* (my school, the school that masters the weapon heart) a modern equivalent of the ancient path, and the Japanese and Chinese authorities that regulate such matters agree with me.

Assuming "the position" and going within to confront or search for the true self from the viewpoint of a psychologist requires courage as well as skill. Each of us can only testify to our own experience or bear witness to the experiences of others. The psychological discoveries can be described in narrative, and that may encourage those who have not yet undertaken the journey of self-transformation. The following is a description drawn from my own experiences as well as those of others focusing on the psychological aspects of transcendental change. (In the chapter entitled "The Kundalini Experience" I describe it from a feeling or sensory perspective.) This description also points out what I perceive to be ends, although the process is not over, as I'm still alive and in this body most of the time.

Let us first suppose that what we consider our self seems to be more a collection of masks or theatrical roles that we present to others. When we explore beneath these sweaty masks we find more masks. Images of what we're supposed to be but no feeling of who we are. These comprise self-image or can be thought of as social roles. We might discover that our impulses toward achievement and compassion spring from a fear of failure and feelings of helplessness. As we plunge deeper we may be forced to discover that these social strivings are but acceptable covers for anger, resentment and envy, leading to undermining of others in the guise of helping them in "friendly competition." Suppose we recognize and take ownership of this sly rage and allow ourselves to open even further to find shame, yearning, terror, sadness, and other dark emotions we normally do not hold to our credit. Often the recognition and controlling of these powerful emotions is considered enough for the adventurer, as he or she quickly sees the advantage of having them under control, particularly where many others do not even seem to realize that they are driven by a darker desire.

Finally suppose when we accept our shadow self and work through to the roots of these turbulent emotions, we find another layer of calm connectedness that allows loving interaction with others without the marked manipulation and ambivalence discovered in our earlier self-reflection. This open acceptance of self and others is utterly different in feeling and context than where we started. Little change may be visible, but you will feel the difference.

It is on the basis of such a narrative that people seek therapy because those of us who have lived it or guided others through it know the value of inner peace and being in touch with the true animal nature, which is fundamentally benevolent and caring. This can be accomplished through years of analysis or more quickly with the guidance of a skilled therapist. You can do it yourself through Zen meditation in three to eight years of *sesshins* (ritualized meditations sitting under the supervision of a Zen *roshi* or meditation master).

Let us suppose that by going into this primal self we find skills and connections not required by life in the polis. Let us suppose that when we are truly relaxed and have removed the masks and barriers to our being what we are rather than what we supposed we were, we find connections beyond the ground of self that force us to reevaluate reality as we once perceived it. With a little study we may find that others have penetrated these inner and outer terrains and based on their honest and diligent exploration have left maps but in a strange language—discussions of endless bliss, energy beings, chakras, lights as a thousand stars, merging with gods, *etcetera ad infinitum.*

One who has experienced love will not find much sympathy when explaining his or her viewpoint to those whose only joy comes from revenge and who find strength in their ability to hate. Thus it is often hard to translate the directions and warnings given by the ancients, as the meanings of the descriptions may have more distance than mere age. You have to go yourself. Sometimes the self-adventurer discovers the truly rare and extraordinary. One who claims to know the way but has not made the journey is neither a good guide nor a complete human being.

Sometimes, as in the case of Aleister Crowley or others who have taken this route in order to achieve dominance or power over others, they find themselves immersed in an overwhelming sadness which is their true self's recognition of their longing for the universal and simultaneous awareness of being alone. The aloneness is a recognition of one's separateness from others and one's place in the cosmos. That too must be questioned and explored. Suppose that as a creature of energy and wavelength and constant change one discovers a new relationship that also contains the material relationship with the world which is universal. Life is a simple presence we all share with each other. When we can appreciate our aloneness we can be ourselves and give most fully, as we no longer need others to save us or make us or reflect us or make us feel good about ourselves. Instead, we want them to become themselves more fully. In this way conscious love is created from the exploration and opening of one's own heart through diligent meditation and introspection. It is only through knowing yourself that true love and compassion evolve. Remember Socrates' dictum, "Know Thyself!" For the martial artist this process is physical as well as psychological/spiritual. The ninja's heart is under the sword, which tends to speed the process if you can relax and trust the sword wielder.

As you study the literature left by the great martial artists of the East, there is always reference to a number of concepts that may seem strange to Western eyes, particularly when after what seem to be stupendous physical exploits, someone says something like "and then I learned about chi kung and really began to learn and understand what I was doing." Chi kung is the training of internal energy through breathing techniques that enhance and change the character of the physical body. It requires total relaxation and calm and results in extraordinary speed, strength, and control. It is the internal key to the external power and the best explanation of why in the internal arts the most dangerous practitioners are usually in their fifties and sixties, whereas those who rely on physical skill alone seldom survive into the thirties regardless of their skills. The practice of chi kung (or Taoist esoteric yoga) when combined with Zen meditation results in the kundalini if done religiously for thirty to ninety days. The end mental product or psychological result seems remarkably similar to what we in the West identify with creative genius and preternatural physical skills if you have properly prepared your body for the onslaught of living energy and hormones. If you don't know what you are doing, it is more like what is described by Gopi Krishna or Christina Grof—eight to twenty years of hell until you give up your fear and grow up.

Most religious traditions have lost the power to the frauds, and most martial arts have been oversold by the ignorant and the sports buffs, but the Way is the same as it always has been for the intelligent who wish to transcend their socially learned self. It is a simple step-by-step process of continuing practice that accumulates like step functions in mathematics. The results of the process can be seen, felt, and tasted. The following are not drawn from the historical record but are empirical descriptions drawn from my own experience, the observations of my students, and verifications by others who have had similar experience of living energy.

Physical characteristics of a true kundalini survivor, *tatsujin*, or complete human being which cannot be faked include:

1. An inch or more of glowing corona around the body that is particularly evident and bright radiating around the head. The completed product is white. No other color need apply. This can be seen against plain backgrounds and most easily in subdued light. For the wearer of a halo, it feels like wearing a cap. Before the energy reaches the head and while it primarily rests in other locations, the corona will be the color usually associated with the organs in Chinese medicine or chakras in the Indian nomenclature for the endocrine system. Each color has distinct personality characteristics or survival mechanisms which can be considered biological. Color also identifies where the energy is held, which could be considered a sign of progress or an indicator of where the energy is blocked. Each chakra is associated with two or more inner deities in the Taoist, Mikkyo Buddhist, and Tibetan systems.

2. The breath is slow, usually four breaths a minute unless one smokes which may up it to six. A nonsmoker from a smog-free area might have a cycle of one or two breaths per minute. The highly skilled can fake death. Both chi kung and the kundalini lead to extremely efficient metabolisms. I've seen this discussed as "the meditator uses less air." It is more accurate to say the medi-

tator uses air with exceptional efficiency and is seldom breathless unless exercising heavily.

3. The saliva is sweet to the taste like honey, thus the reference to nectar of the gods across cultures, and it flows freely resulting in better digestion and disease control. This is a result of the energizing of the brain stem and pituitary.

4. The heart rate is quite slow and the body temperature remains below normal. Gopi Krishna's heart rate remained high as a stress reaction; he was scared and with good reason. Blood pressure may be lower depending on personal habits.

5. The musculature is soft and very supple, more like an athletic girl than a man, which is probably a by-product of the rejuvenation of the endocrine system and accounts for the association with androgyny. This is what Okinawan practitioners of karate refer to when they describe the body of a master as "steel wrapped in cotton." The bones appear harder and whiter under X-ray. The mental linking of intention with action backed by the endocrine system often results in what is perceived by the more hesitant as superhuman strength and speed.

6. Close association with one of these complete human beings will kick your body's electrical system into overdrive. Their very presence raises most peoples' excitement levels, so they're fun to party with. You feel strange when they're around until you get used to them, unless they've learned to hide their *wa* (harmonious spirit), as taught in some Japanese martial arts associated with the gathering of intelligence. Often this feeling of higher energy results in sexual arousal and can be mildly embarrassing if your teacher is of the same gender and not inclined or vice versa. (Higher energy is also sexual energy.) My son informs me that just being in the same house with me kicks in his adrenals. You easily feel people with chi, and people without active chi are very difficult to sense by comparison. Feelings may also be exchanged, which may be perceived as radical mood shifts when you enter into the survivor's range. The kundalini survivor learns to stay in neutral so as not to wreak havoc on his or her friends. The power of this energy does not seem to fade but continually increases

with use. The more I do, the stronger I get, the better I feel. This also seems true of every practitioner of chi kung that I know. This higher energy accelerates healing of self and others. Cuts and scratches heal in days. Most diseases that are not virus-linked no longer affect one, and flu symptoms, are minimized.

7. Body movement is very controlled, as the integration of mind, body and spirit results in an ability to move with great speed out of complete stillness. There is no thinking involved, just action in response to action. This is not a result of programming but is creative response. To the observer it is very fluid and graceful, not robotic or mechanical. The whole body is involved, not just an arm or a leg. It is hard to describe, but once seen is never forgotten. A policeman I train with occasionally described me as going from completely relaxed, to completely on, to completely relaxed in the same second, which he felt was very "spooky." Personally, I find uptight, perfectionist, hard-bodied people much more spooky.

8. There is surprising strength regardless of size, which usually takes a while to master. One has a tendency to break things until one learns to lighten up. I went through a period of breaking keys off in locks, ripped the handle off a car door one icy morning, and sent many of my students screaming to the floor until I learned to slow down and back off. Some of the ninjas I play with call me Dr. Death. Even affectionate squeezes and hugs are not appreciated, and love-making can be filled with minor perils if the object of your affection does not share your rare affliction or athleticism. One of my shodan, Bret Talbot, ran up a considerable lab bill in broken beakers while working on chemistry projects. He claims he was only holding them gently in his hands when they imploded. He still thinks he is gentle when he is dangerous as a bear. You have to be careful with this strange strength. The feeling is invincibility, but the reality still won't stop bullets.

9. The *tatsujin* or complete human being is calm and balanced under most conditions. Physical balance is one-pointed in that the center flows to the grounded point. The center is mobile, which makes for a strange three-dimensionality of movement,

something like a dancer or gymnast but not as athletic or aesthetic in appearance. Folk as opposed to ballet. A master boxer can fight balanced on one leg. Shiva stands one-footed on the dwarf of ignorance. To be completely honest you may want to observe apes and monkeys and then draw your own conclusions in terms of natural body movement. All the masters and myself included move like monkeys, which can be very amusing. The study of yoga provides a graceful, uplifting balance. Androgyny can also be seen as balanced.

10. There is a tenth characteristic that is seen more in the religious than the martial practitioner. Georg Feurstein alludes to it in his book *Holy Madness,* which is an excellent exposition of Crazy Wisdom that shares some of the same characteristics of divine madness exhibited by Zen-oriented martial practitioners. The characteristic of knowing from many subtle inputs does have the effect of distancing one from what is observed. The religious practitioner has to deal with converts who see transformation as a mental process instantaneously accomplished. They know better but are trapped by socially learned expectations. It is difficult to continually forgive and suffer fools. Losing one's objectivity, however, usually creates even greater difficulties. Karma.

The above are the primary physical symptoms of the complete and safe transforming by the kundalini, which is greatly aided by the safer technology of chi kung. This is actually a biological process available to anyone who meditates and masters the techniques for moving sexual energy through the microcosmic orbits. Knowing the technology of awakening the inner self removes most of the physiological dangers. A guru or *Oshihan* should manifest all these characteristics both mental and physical, as they are the same for both sexes and a result of connecting the meridians and rejuvenating the endocrine system.

When I took Suzanne Carlson, my first female shodan in twenty years of teaching, through the kundalini in London, the only after-effect was permanently dilated eyes, which is not exactly a disadvantage when you're an actress. She ran bliss for a couple of hours and reported "seeing" with the third eye a scorpion, then a fox's skull, and then a smile or half moon tilted to the side as is usually shown on the forehead of Diana the huntress or the goddess Athena or Egypt's Nepthys. One should not expect ovarian energy to have exactly the same symbolism for the brain as testicular. Her father asked her if she were on drugs when he saw her eyes a couple of days later. She went through a brief period of feeling very superior as her psychic abilities manifested, and like Gurdjieff noticed practically everyone she knew seemed half asleep or were simply rats in a maze having no control over their lives or desires. She went through a brief period of testing her fearlessness by trying out dangerous practices. Then like most of us who have done this, she reacquired humility and got on with creating her life and career.

We followed Mantak Chia's instructions concerning not allowing hot energy to enter the skull until the way is prepared including the practice of keeping the tongue up. The female experience is similar to the male's but with the usual differences rooted in our biological nature. Some of the ancient Taoists wrote that women were incapable of chi generation. The Roman Catholic Church forbids the ordination of priestesses. A fox skull has the same outline as the two ovaries and vessels leading to the uterus and vagina, as does the arc of the browed moon or the raised tail of the scorpion—all symbolic of bringing female sexual energy to the forehead up the spine. Suzanne is the only woman I've been privileged to observe go through the kundalini. We were able to discuss what was happening when she came down, and it was great fun. We had to run out to the West End and buy a copy of Cooper's *Illustrated Encyclopedia of Traditional Symbols* to keep abreast.

Kammy, a female friend of Mike Cornelius reported a blindingly bright yellow banana shape appearing as her solar plexus opened. She is running very hot energy now when she used to run cold. I know two other young women who developed all the energy characteristics of the *lesser kan and li* but have not had the experience of ovary-to-brain connection via the spinal column. Blake Poindexter has specialized in training women. We are both of the opinion that women are easier to teach and develop more power than men. It is probably the reason some of the ancients forbade the teaching of women. It's terribly embarrassing to be thrown about physically and mentally by a woman, even when you love her. It's easier to maintain a master/slave relationship. Very few of the ancients seemed to follow the example of the Yellow Emperor, who kept and learned from his female companions.

The martial artist who becomes involved in physical transformation that results in transpersonal growth tends not to lose his or her sense of humor. We also realize that once the typical seeker sees our path, they look for something less risky. We know that most not only won't but can't get IT. We tend to let our student/victim/client/friends struggle through the belt system at their own speed or drive them away if they can't develop higher expectations. It is a tragedy from my viewpoint that our institutions burdened with the role of leading us to enlightenment are failing us due to fear and ignorance. It is sad indeed when martial artists can demonstrate greater effect than ministers and priests. Study on this.

Chapter Three

The Kundalini Experience

BEING A COLLEGE PROFESSOR means you have the summer off to indulge in little self-improvement projects. When the school year ended in 1985 I decided to follow the prescriptions given in my chi kung correspondence course from the Chinese National Chi Kung Institute in Moulton, Alabama, to arouse the bubbling springs or bring the inner fire to the brain. This is known as Tien Tao Chi Kung or Heaven's Way and corresponds to the Indian Kundalini. I'd been able to run the microcosmic orbit connecting the meridians and chakras to the spine both front and back with a single breath for about three years and was able to bend a candle flame to my bidding, so I thought I'd go for the big time. Ninety days of meditating as much as possible.

I set up a pad in the back porch and moved in a stereo tape player so I could meditate to ragas, Kitaro, or subliminals (which I recommend if you're nutso enough to try this method). My second wife Linda and her children would occasionally look out from the kitchen to see what I was doing. Since watching someone meditate ranks in spectator sports right down there with spider kissing, they failed to get involved. The back porch was my kingdom for the summer as long as I occasionally got up to eat, take them to the lake, and performed as a parent and husband. Otherwise I sat cross-legged, listening to funny music with my eyes shut. After all, her first husband used to beat her and them. My activities seemed strange but harmless. They did their things and I did mine.

At this point in my development I was not particularly nocturnal so I always meditated in the daytime (my first error). I would hit the position for at least thirty minutes on waking and set my goals for the day. Some days I would get in an hour or two in the morning and another hour or so in the afternoon. About twenty days into it I began to see what appeared to be a vagina with a rather swollen clitoris floating in the air before me. I took this as a sign that the pineal and pituitary glands in the brain were rejuvenating and/or the third eye was opening. Some days I would sweat profusely as I meditated, which I regarded as a good sign because it indicated something was happening. It is not usual to break into a fever-busting sweat when you're being absolutely still, at least not in my mediocre athletic career. Sweating is both a means to cool the inner fire as well as a process of purification. That's why sweat lodges, saunas, and hot baths are appreciated. My body was starting to feel great and I was horny as a three-peckered owl. This is where I made my second mistake, which would eventually cost me this marriage.

Let me digress for a moment and set the scene. I weighed about 240 pounds, smoked a pack or more of filter tips a day, enjoyed wine with my meals, ate a lot of red meat, and preferred Rusty Nails (Scotch and Drambuie 50/50, no ice) as my daily libation. When I meditated I did not usually keep my tongue up, as I could not see how that could be important. I was not properly stretching my neck but had mastered holding my back erect. I was 41 years old, succumbing to a potbellied, sedentary middle age. The only redeeming factor was I worked out with my martial arts class once a week for an hour or two, which kept my reflexes quick and was restoring my body after eight years of being a scholarly, deskbound wimp.

I want to be perfectly clear that the kundalini is not a result of perfect asanas, *ahimsa* (nonviolence) and a vegetarian diet, which are logical progressions resulting from the experience but have little or nothing to do with attaining it. My practice was directed toward perfecting iron palm techniques, and I wanted enough voltage to shatter concrete blocks without effort or harm to myself. I certainly wasn't celibate and, until the first great disaster, Linda and I had a varied and active sex life, as we both considered sex the best form of exercise.

I was feeling like a twenty-year-old, semi-erect all the time. I decided to masturbate, put some porn on the VCR, and was beating off while standing. Suddenly a tremendous burst of energy ripped up my back and hit the base of my skull. The pain was so intense I fell to my knees. I wanted to vomit. The back of my neck began to burn along with my right elbow, which I'd injured doing stupid tae kwan do katas a few years back and then reinjured playing tennis. From that day for the next six months sex was not a pleasure, as from the moment of erection I'd become nauseated and every stroke was a race to see if I'd faint or throw up from pain. Orgasm was a relief, but attaining it was a superhuman effort. I tried to explain what was happening to Linda but she wasn't buying into it. Actions spoke much louder than words. All she could see was my struggle and, not having the highest self-esteem, decided I either hated making love to her or had taken a mistress and now found her repugnant. Fighting this kind of pain and keeping an erection was not easy. She asked for a divorce. I gave her the house, cars, set up trusts for her kids, and went adventuring.

Chi sickness or emerging kundalini problems weren't part of her perceptual world or mine. Fortunately Dr. Richard Grant, a political economist at the college who was taking my hoshinjutsu course, had read in the field of Ayurvedic medicine and recommended Mantak Chia's work to me. The techniques of Taoist esoteric yoga corresponded to the chi kung but had some additional safety factors built in such as stronger emphasis on keeping one's tongue up when meditating as well as reversing the direction of the energy occasionally when running the microcosmic orbit. I was eventually able to heal the damage done to the *jade gates* (energy

31

entry points) at the base of my skull and return to a normal sex life but the damage to my marriage was irredeemable. It wasn't until after Linda divorced me and finally developed her own chi through transmission that she was able to swallow that whopper.

At this point there was nothing to do but press on. I continued my practice even though it was painful. Some part of me knew I had to continue or lose all that I felt I had gained. The spectral clitoral vagina still floated before me. I realized the cause of my problem probably also contained the cure. When I wasn't meditating I became an avid researcher in esoteric literature and transpersonal psychology. About forty days in, my body began to shake as soon as I hit the position that is often referred to as the half-lotus or sage seat. I have never been able to sit in full lotus with any comfort, and at this time my ankles were not stretched enough to hold in *seiza* for the required time periods. Once the shaking started, things really began to get strange. This was the beginning of bliss.

Now, I wasn't keeping a record of these events, as I didn't realize the importance of what I was doing. To me it was just a way to improve my martial art. I'd attended two of Stephen Hayes' *Go Dai* (five centers) seminars and been impressed by what I'd seen and done with the ninjas. It had also struck me as funny that most of the people I knew studied Eastern philosophy but did not practice what they were studying. Theirs was an intellectual, not a physical involvement. And to be quite frank, becoming a guru or Hare Krishna or cult member struck me as the ultimate in silliness. I had stayed away from the religious aspects as I was quite content being a failed Methodist and still feel that way except for occasional excursions into goddess worship. My concerns were purely technical and my expectations were to gain control over my body's electrical system. I can't give an exact chronology of the following events as they seemed not to be consecutive but concurrent. Anyway, what happened was totally unexpected.

About the middle of July, close to my birthday, the floating vagina turned into a tiny dancer of Balinese extraction and zoomed up to me on one foot and hovered in the air in front of me. I was flabbergasted. I was having hallucinations of Hindu temple whores? She stood on one foot with her arms spread wide wearing a metal breastplate, pointy helmet, and funny flared miniskirt. My impression at the time was this apparition was female and, for some reason unknown to me, was telling me to put more dance into my training. I perceived that the spread arms meant, "See, I have the big head, graceful movement is important." It wasn't until years later that I realized this was Shiva, the destroyer of the ego (or ignorance). My latent homophobia kept me from realizing the androgyny of this personage, and my ignorance of Hindu religion left me with no recourse but to watch this improbable vision as it watched me. I suspect we were both equally surprised. I don't know how long this went on. I was frozen in place for quite a while.

Years later when Suzanne and I were playing in the Victoria and Albert Museum in London, I saw a statue of Shiva and this piece of the puzzle fell into place. Ah well, I missed my chance to speak with a god. Shiva's posture is similar to *Hicho no Kamae* (karate kid's white crane) in ninjutsu.

The next event was more physical. As I was running energy around the orbit and looking and smiling down into myself and shaking with energy, I saw a brownish-gold coil of powerful energy building at the base of my spine. It had a head like a viper and began to come up my spinal column. As it hit each vertebrae it would straighten and adjust it, throwing me from side to side. The feeling was of being slammed about but I never came off the *zafu*. This was terrifying, particularly after the penis-migraine-nausea hookup. I was lost. Nothing I had ever read prepared me for this. It was inside me. God damn these chi kung exercises! I could see it coming with my inner eye like a freight train coming up a tunnel, and when it reached the skull this time there was no mercy and no stopping it.

My head exploded. It was as if the top of my skull blew off and I was radiating up into a fountain of white light. Then I was white light. I wasn't just sitting on the back porch, I was part of the house and the yard and the trees and the birds and the grass and the cat and it all made sense from an evolutionary perspective as

33

my consciousness rocketed out of Jonesville, Michigan, into universal ecstasy. Darwin was right. It's survival of the fittest, but fit has many meanings and everything is connected to everything on an atomic level; the whole has a spirit or direction that might be defined as God, or energy, or self/creativity if you're inclined in that direction. The messages I was getting made no sense in terms of good or bad. It was just here it is and you're part of it and it's part of you, and though you're a small part, you can affect the whole. Do your best as you're on your own. Krishnamurti describes a very similar experience as does Gopi Krishna.

As this experience was winding down, my life began to pass before my eyes as if I were watching a movie running backwards in slow motion. I got to watch how I'd screwed up important relationships and what lessons I'd learned or failed to learn in my interactions with others. Most of the important learnings took place when I was very young. Like the song goes, "Teach your children well."

The wildest memory was of being sperm. Even sperm has consciousness. How's this for a lesson: I was racing down a tunnel toward a pink light. I was part of a horde of little lights who were also me, and we were all trying to reach the big pink first. It was imperative, as the goal was attractive. The race was close and we/me were all going at top speed. I/me/we hit the pink first. Another we/me was right behind me by a millisecond. I watched it die with all the other we/mes as I merged with the pink. That's my first lucid memory. Now the lesson from this could be all organisms have consciousness and should be treated as part of the holy spirit. I think my particular interpretation ran more like winning is real important, which I suspect is the more usual outcome for men from this deep-seated universal experience. How one is raised would definitely reinforce either interpretation.

The memories stopped at conception, no past lives. No womb swimming. No birthing experience. When I saw the opening to the movie *Look Who's Talking* years later I almost fell out of the seat laughing. Since death is as universal as life, this memory cannot be sentimentalized into an argument against abortion. An ant has the same relation to intelligence or problem-solving. Sentience is not the same as existence. I can't buy into "every sperm is sacred," as my tendencies are definitely hedonistic. The food chain exists.

This whole thing was stretching to the limit what my first wife, Martha, used to refer to as "your fucking Zen Buddhist calm!" There weren't any stress management techniques for dealing with these life events. And the dance had only just begun. I was still locked in position, morning had come and gone as a still, small voice began to speak to me. "Oh, your neck hurts; well, look at your eyelids." I could see a holograph of my skull and neck bones as if it were an X-ray, except when I moved my head the holograph replicated the movement. "See the damage here. That's high school football, and this one, that's karate. Now stick out your arm, turn your hand over and shift your shoulder this way." The vertebrae slipped into place easily and a residual pain that I'd been ignoring for twenty years went away. "Now isn't that nice. Why don't you just let me take over. I know how to take care of this body."

Whoa, this was getting a little too strange even for me. I'd seen *The Exorcist*. What was going on now? Voices in my head! "Get thee behind me, Satan!" Which is one of Jesus's better puns when you know about the spine. Who do you call, Ghostbusters?

An interesting debate ensued as to who owned what. The id had now emerged and proceeded to show the learned personality which I still perceived as me what was what. "You think what you see is real, try this."

The back porch became a forest, my meditating pillow a rock. I could hear birds singing as the wind moved the branches of the trees. I was naked, the sun was going down. "I'm your body," the voice said, "I process everything that you see, hear, feel, or do. You don't know what's real. I do." I was back on the pillow facing into the kitchen, considerably shaken.

"Look," I said, "I'm a college professor. For all I know, you're not even housebroken. You may be able to run this body, but how are your lecture skills? I have to feed my family. Let's make a deal. I mean we're both me. How can we merge?"

What happened next I can only describe as a fist being shoved through another fist, but it was taking place in my skull. My perceptions were going through some very interesting changes and my body began to change. Some of those changes are still going on today, which is about eight years later. As the inner voice quieted, I asked one more question. "What would you have done if I hadn't opted for merger?"

The voice grew large, seemed to come from all around me, and said, "I am a jealous God and will have no other gods before me! Obey me and live according to my custom!" A very interesting support for bicameral brain theory. Then it went, "If you didn't go for that, there is always something like this . . . I'm Xantha, a 10,000-year-old warrior from Atlantis. Allow me to enter through you and share the learning of the ages." That seemed to take care of channels. If you don't allow the learned personality (ego and/or superego) to die when you meditate, the id will try to fool you into letting it run the body. That was the last time "the spirit" spoke as a separate entity.

Chi sickness is a result of the body's inability to process higher energy or move it from place to place by the direction of the imagination. The Taoist traditions place great emphasis on *wa* (harmony). Moving the energy through the microcosmic and macrocosmic orbits accomplishes this mixing to help achieve inner harmony. As one's internal wattage increases it is often described as "inner fire" or "fire in the belly" since excess energy can be stored in the intestinal coil or *hara*. The object of Taoist meditation is to bring the fire to the brain and then through the rest of the body. Wherever the nerve synapses are not flexible enough to handle the voltage there can be considerable pain. Eventually the body will adjust to the energy if your practice allows you to move it. It is important to realize that chi moves most easily in circles and spirals. It is also important to know that the yang energy burns, while the yin energy cools. The cooling heals the burning. Running hot yang energy is easy for most males and many women. One imagines the cycle at first, but when the real thing begins you will instantly know the difference. Running cool yin energy is difficult as it is usually produced by the left side of the body, which right-handers allow to atrophy.

It took me years of study after going through the kundalini to get even sporadic control of cool energy until Suzanne Carlson mastered it while studying dance, acting, and celibacy in London. She called me from England and told me she had been running icy cold energy for days and it was scaring her as she couldn't get it under control. By the time I got to London she had figured it out and could contain the phenomenon. She had a lot of fun showing me how. Toffesse (who is described in the "Exchanges with Interesting People" chapter) could change from yin to yang on command but never could explain how he was doing it. Suzanne, being brilliant, articulate, and in touch with her body and spirit, was able to pass on this skill necessary for higher-level healing. I've been cool for five years now.

From 1986 through 1988 my body went through extremely painful sessions of what I refer to as rewiring. When the stomach rewired there was a period of three days that I could keep down no food or water. The pain was intense, but as all medical tests showed absolutely nothing, I knew I'd have to ride it out. I'd drink a glass or two of water to keep dehydration at a minimum and then run to kneel at the shrine of the porcelain god when it came back up. This was a continual ritual. Once when the urge to upchuck was upon me and I was getting out of the easy chair to make the scramble down the hall to the bathroom, my eyes turned off.

My immediate thought was, "Oh, no! I'm going to be blind!" I still had to throw up, so I crawled down the hall feeling my way as fast as I could. Being blind is one thing, barfing all over Linda's living room is quite another. As I fired into the toilet, feeling quite pleased with myself for conquering this first obstacle with my new challenge or handicap, my eyes turned back on. That has never happened since. But other interesting rewires seem to take place at odd moments when you've nothing better to do. Your whole body will eventually rewire and some parts are definitely not as much fun as others. Every place you've been seriously injured, had a bone broken, or taken some nerve damage will receive special attention, as damage improperly healed often creates a block to the efficient flow of energy. Blocked higher energy burns! Those areas referred to as erogenous zones tend to hold one's attention when they light up. It never seems to happen when you're driving or doing anything dangerous. (It also seems to happen again every few years.) If you've managed to poison yourself, it can be much like an epileptic seizure. Your social mind shuts down, you sweat copiously, empty at both ends, and in minutes feel great. Not a pretty sight but better than being poisoned. I've had that experience three times. Chi allows you to drink enormous amounts of alcohol but the poison eventually wins.

Most of my students who kept their tongues up when running the orbits had much gentler experiences of the kundalini than I. A female diabetic in Fenton, Michigan, informs me her pancreas now produces insulin after being shut off for fifteen years. She went through some weeks of barfing and is now on soups and yogurt. Her name is Laura Butler, and she designs custom fantasy jewelry. She decorated my sword scabbard with Chinese-Japanese monsters that are associated with enlightenment.

It took me over five years to rewire the damage done when the first rush of kundalini energy hit the Jade Gates and couldn't get through to the brain. That area on the back of the head is always the first to inform me when it's time to visit the chiropractor or get back to my neck stretches. It seems to me the process is much easier if you're in good shape. I was not. I'm in much better shape now than I was in my twenties. When I went through the kundalini I was fat and degenerate; now I'm much slimmer and more circumspect in my diet. Suppleness is critical! Gopi Krishna almost died. Krishnamurti had relatively few problems (and hid his sexuality) but had the support of the Theosophist movement. Alexander the Great fell down and foamed from time to time. Hatsumi says he went through a period of grave illness where nothing he knew seemed to work anymore. He had to live on yogurt for eighteen months. Can you even imagine what that would do to a Grandmaster's ego? This can be dangerous if you miss some of the parts.

According to the transpersonal psychologists who research in this area, most of the people go through spiritual crises and the ones who have a full-blown kundalini experience tend to retire from society. I can understand why. Things get strange and you have no one to share your experience. Visual and auditory hallucinations or strange energy rushing through the body, were seldom discussed in my circle of friends. Prolonged altered states that do not go away are hard to explain when you do know what's going on! One kundalini survivor I interviewed went for more than twenty years without saying a thing about it until he met me, as he had no idea why he was the way he was, only that he was radically different in his perceptions and much smarter, stronger, and faster than anyone he knew. He did not even discuss it with his wife or family. He had constructed a very comfortable life but was without friendship.

The Pathway or routes to enlightened survival recommended by Sun Tzu are similar in attitude if not practice to the *avadhuta*. They allow one to be active in both worlds. Being fearless means no inhibitions. The enlightened invariably have a childlike earthy quality. When you first pass through the veil, there is a strong tendency to feel very superior to all the people you know who haven't done this. It shouldn't last too long. Your taijutsu skills may improve just from net dodging. Invisibility is more secure than invincibility, as you'll discover. The general population's expectations don't include this form of adventure as entertainment, and the elite do their level-headed best to stamp it out. Be careful.

People like to be the way they are and it is not for you to mess with them. You'll have enough problems dealing with what life throws at you. We're all in this together. Anyone is capable of doing chi kung to achieve the kundalini but there are definite dues and you will pay them. You pass through hell to achieve heaven. The Gods do indeed check you out. There are some very lively "concepts" or "archetypes" that seem to enjoy hanging out around you that can only be logically explained in religious terms and the presence of some rather atypical but archaic ideas. The best all-around general advice I found to go along with "Love thy neighbor as you would love thyself" and "Do unto others as you would have them do unto you" is this short list of maxims by the Gautama Buddha in his Sutra to the Kalamas:

> Do not believe in anything simply because you have heard (or read) it.
>
> Do not believe in traditions because they have been handed down for many generations.
>
> Do not believe in anything because it is spoken and rumored by many.
>
> Do not believe in anything simply because it is written in your religious books.
>
> Do not believe in anything merely on the authority of your teachers and elders.
>
> but
>
> After observation and analysis, when you find anything that agrees with reason and is conducive to the good and benefit of one and all, then accept it and live up to it.

Some of the changes since those days: I no longer follow a regimen of daily meditation but seem to be in a relaxed state nearly all the time. I no longer fear death or any other thing. I am absolutely convinced that if you kill another human being for any reason, you'll be back here. "Here" is not always what we think it is and your condition may not be optimal. (Dante could never have imagined a bag lady in the Bronx.) My senses have become very acute, particularly at night. I'm more empathic and on rare occasions telepathic, both of which I regard as an aid to compassion and a pain in the ass. I'm continually horrified by how people justify their treatment of each other. I have very few friends my own age, though most people seem to like me. I seldom get sick. I do occasionally get damaged, which I'll describe in the chapter on Screwing Up, along with other reasons your relation with the medical doctors can get to be high-risk. I weep and laugh easily. Major sporting events used to reduce me to an emotional moron as I would be literally swept up by the emotions of the crowd even though I seldom care who wins. I will only attend rock concerts with trusted friends. Music and crowds just amplify chi. I have a wonderful time.

I can affect others' energy fields at will. Anyone who gets within thirty feet of me can be affected with ease. My curiosity concerning the human predicament is boundless, but my interest in technology is medieval. Learning to use a Mac was a struggle, but I love computers now. Immediately after going through the kundalini experience I found it very difficult to read. A page or two a day was exhausting. I now read a book a week, but I used to read a book a day and once even taught speed reading when I was in graduate school. The spirit is nonverbal! Everyone I know who practices chi kung goes through a period of reading difficulty. If you like to read the skill comes back. Your taste in literature may change.

I no longer work for anyone I do not like, and I base that on feeling. (Goodbye to wealth.) Most of the religious writings with the exception of Patanjali strike me as poppycock. They describe the life, but not the practice that resulted in the life. Religious writers tend to gloss over the schizophrenia or epilepsy or other fun characteristics of being "touched by God" and not being able to bear the voltage. Only Gopi Krishna and Krishnamurti's descriptions seem to parallel my own, and I find it interesting that an agnostic Westerner following Chinese medical practice would have Hindu experiences. It is obviously biological and has nothing to do with culture, religion, or racial grouping. The only enlightened people I've met (and I can count them on my fingers) have been martial artists, a young Zen monk, healers, and the Dalai Lama. If you take offense at this, I will thank you to note my father was a Methodist minister on the World Council of Evangelism and I've a wide acquaintance of Christians of various stripe. My standards are primarily bioelectrical. Your standards are yours. I am not inclined to worship. I enjoy working out and beating up young people.

I continue to practice and teach the martial arts, as it is a nonreligious and relatively easy way of passing on this knowledge. You have to do it! Reading about it is just looking at the map, or pointing at the moon. Good works may or may not teach you compassion. Sit zazen and learn to breathe using chi kung methodology, get into yoga to stretch out your spine and learn balance, go dancing and fall in love, and do something really scary for focus and hormones—real combatic martial arts, mountain climbing, performing arts, open sea scuba diving, hunting beasties with primitive weapons or humans, or hardest of all, make a new friend. All tend to focus one's creative potential and desire to live.

Arousal is critical to growth, change, and love. Most important, keep your tongue up. When you've finally got IT or merged with your nature, the commonest phosphorescent holographs on your eyelids will look like the Rose Window in Notre Dame, as well as other shapes alluded to in mystical records, such as the lotus rooted in the mud and floating on the water. It does not seem reasonable to me that the old mystical saw concerning "as the inside, so the outside" can be reversed by staring at mandalas, but the iconic similarities are probably meant as guides. One of the things that always annoyed me about the Rajneesh and others of his ilk was they had the order of the colors wrong.

The kundalini has legendary counterparts in Gothic, Greek, American Indian, Celtic, Chinese, Hindu, Japanese, African, Hawaiian, and other mythologies. This cross-cultural commonality strongly indicates it is a universal human experience. References to the snake wisdom or kundalini are usually designated as demonic or evil in Christian mythology referencing the Garden of Eden. It must be recognized, however, that the gift of the serpent was knowledge. It is knowledge that leads us to the life of adventure. Just as the spider has the dual meaning of creator of the universe as well as the web of illusion, the coiled serpent signifies the cycles of manifestation as well as latent power. Coiled around a tree or any axial symbol, the serpent represents the dynamic force or genius of all growing things. Genius means genii or spirit or *kami* (Japanese spirit of a particular place) and may also represent a skill. Associated with the tree of knowledge it is identified as evil by Christians, yet when associated with the tree of life the same serpent is regarded as beneficial. The horned serpent or dragon or serpent-wreathed head are universally regarded as symbols of fertility and creativity as well as an intermediary to the gods.

Kundalini as a means and outcome of mastering energy is an actual biological process that when observed objectively closely follows its mythic description. J. C. Cooper defines it as "the serpent which lies coiled at the base of the spine in the chakra known as the *muladhara* [the Japanese like *hara*] and which lies dormant until awakened by yogic and spiritual practices when it begins to ascend through the *chakras* [endocrine glands or Go Dai], bringing increasing powers into play, until it reaches the highest point in total awareness and realization. It is latent energy; unawakened being; the sleeping serpent power; the primordial *shakti* [creative female energy] in man. To awaken it is to break the ontological plane and attain the sacred Center: enlightenment. The symbolism of the kundalini is associated with that of the serpent, or dragon, or spine, the world axis."

This is not trivial knowledge, nor is it evil, though enlightened common men have always been feared by the established order particularly if it has lost its Way. This is worth setting some time aside to attempt. My experience and observations lead me to assert that you should clean up your act before seriously starting the meditative process. It is also helpful if you have some interesting life experience under your belt or your IQ is well above average, as the gods are real when you enter the void and they will test your endurance. There is interesting work to be done.

Chapter Four

Traditional Relationships and Teaching in Esoteric Martial Arts

THE PREFERRED, BUT seldom achieved, teaching relationship is one of mutual trust and consulting. I know things you don't know. You know things I don't know. We both benefit from sharing. There is always a hierarchy in experience but with respect it doesn't have to be formalized to any great extent. Distancing creates many problems in communication. All science appears as magic to the ignorant. Ignorance is not stupidity but not learning. In Christian nomenclature, ignorance is missing the mark or "sinning." My father informs me that the word *sin* is a Greek archers' term used when the archer misses the target. The fool killer Kali, the spider goddess, as well as Shiva, balance on the corpse of ignorance. Dr. Norman R. F. Maier (my industrial psychology mentor) said, "The easiest way to identify smart people is to look for who's asking questions."

In the traditional master-student relationship, a master parcels out information and experience according to his or her perception of the student's readiness to receive. Master Sherm Harrill spent years on the karate basics in Okinawa. Shimabuku gave him scrolls when he left for the States. The master had rewarded and recognized his sincerity. It took Sherm years to figure out what he'd been given. It helps to have a translator when you're dealing with the inscrutable. Leo Sebregst's teacher, a retired Chinese general, made him watch for seven years while he tried to teach his own sons. Finally he relented and said, "Since you've shown more interest than they have, come and get it!" or words to that effect. Takamatsu is described by his wife as being delighted with having Hatsumi as a student. At the shidoshi training for godan and above in Noda City, Hatsumi rolled out Takamatsu's scrolls for us to admire and spoke about how often he goes back to read the letters and cards from Takamatsu and returns to the scrolls to discover new insights.

I know from my own experience trying to teach street people what a drain it is to teach those who can't or won't learn. All of my students have confirmed for me how much more fun it is to teach smart people regardless of their physical skills. It's easy to see why Takamatsu would love having Hatsumi for a student. You would give your left nut to teach a real genius, it's so much fun. In expanding our venturesome militaristic societies, the study of unarmed combat is considered in the province of gentlemen. In a democratic, business oriented society, it is too often limited to disciplining children, entertaining adults, or being studied by thugs. It is a lengthy, painful growth process to learn the real thing as the levels of risk and your avoidance skills expand. Neither raw intellect nor great physical skill compare well to the lessons of endurance. The master or guru and disciple or deshi relationship requires deep bonding and closeness. This is a relationship and friendship for life.

When Hatsumi was demoing in Dayton, Ohio, for a Japanese TV network special in the early eighties, I saw his aura running high-voltage green wind chi. He started doing techniques on Steve Hayes, Bud Malmstrom, and Jack Hoban: the looks on their faces as he sent them sailing were an appropriate mix of awe and terror. I loved it when Hatsumi said, "Now my American instructors are at a level where I can use more of my power." Only an outsider with developed chi could really appreciate the looks they gave each other when he said that after what he'd just done to them. It looked like, "Oh, no. It's starting again." Hatsumi's motto is "Keep going. Keep playing." In other words, "Never quit. Have fun. This is your life. Enjoy it."

Ninjo (endurance under the stick? beating emotions into place?) is the concept of human feelings being vastly more important than what is logical and profitable. For the time and effort a sensei invests in a student he hopes the student will realize *tsukiai* (the social debt incurred by the student toward the teacher). Tsukiai in ancient times would manifest itself by the student taking care of the teacher's family, shelter, or whatever he or she needed to be more comfortable. *Giri,* the obligations or debts the student owes to a real shihan, are considered *gimu* (endless), and no matter what is given, it will never be enough for the gift of enlightened life or spirit. Giri to one's associates, however, is repaid according to the significance of the obligation or gift received, and it must be repaid promptly.

The titles of teachers have meaning beyond teacher. *Shihan* means knight/scholar and head of a particular school. *Shi,* referring to four and death, is also Japanese for chi as manifested by spirit. Shihan then has a hidden meaning as one who can give chi. *Shichidan* or seventh degree has three obvious meanings that are concealed from the outsider by using the number designation *nanaedan. Oshihan* is a self-made master in reference to chi, holds no obligations to a teacher, and is able to pass on his skills. It is also a term used to refer to someone who has thousands of followers as head of a particular school. The title is interchangeable in terms of quality or quantity resulting in knowledge lost to popularity. Big organizations often lose their hearts to size.

Amae (unconditional affection) is the core concept of Japanese culture and the foundation of their psyche. For lack of a better definition it could be described as indulgent love. Francis L.K. Hsu wrote an excellent ethnography of Japanese concepts and behavior that I read some twenty years ago and can't remember the title. In Rogerian psychology *amae* would be total acceptance of the other.

Regardless of physical skills, the person with the most experience is regarded as *sempai* (senior) and the person with less experience as *kohai* (heart that says yes? or junior). Sempai have an obligation to develop the kohai. The kohai have an obligation to tend to the needs of the sempai.

Most Americans have no desire to become grown-up dojo boys to a rigidly traditional master. It smacks of indentured servitude and taxation without representation. We are used to receiving public education, and with the exception of apprenticeship avoid in-depth relationships with teachers. We pay them money rather than serve them always. The actual behavior among sempai and kohai, however, is usually of the older indulging the younger to be boisterous and rowdy under the master's protection. The sempai observes from the background while the kohai acts as his or her agent. The sempai will reach out to save the kohai if disaster threatens. The kohai shares a fresh perspective with the sempai which keeps the senior up to date. It's a powerful relationship.

The kohai/sempai relation is supposed to be one of indulgence. The relationships between the ninjas and their American students have to be pretty forgiving, as most people who are drawn to this sort of thing tend to be wild and headstrong (as well as have more redeeming qualities). Often a kohai will be over-promoted by the sempai with the expectation he or she will grow into the new position. After Hatsumi gave me a shidoshi license at godan, I told him if he wanted to protect the ryu's reputation for excellence in taijutsu he had better quit promoting me. Expectations of behavior could be better researched on both sides, but all wounds seem to heal eventually or at least become smoothed over out of curiosity and politeness. In some ways it is like belonging to the tennis league and playing doubles. You get to know people on a number of levels. You are there to learn and play. If you can't handle it, you back off.

Giri can also be translated as discipline, and a discipline requires disciples, which is the term often used in Chinese systems for a student of a chi kung or kung fu master. The Japanese term for a disciple is *deshi*. The relationship is considered religious, for life, and the kung fu or kempo training hall, or kwoon, is a temple. The disciple is often the memory of the master and studies in one particular discipline of a large system. By being the memory of the master, a disciple perfects a particular form and specializes in teaching that part of the system. (I don't cartwheel out of flips, but my student Todd Smith and ninja shihan Greg Kowalski can. If you are athletic enough to want that as part of your response system, you go to Todd for that lesson, as my body tends to fail at that level. You want to learn that technique from someone who does it with grace rather than the hope of avoiding injury. The knights stand in for the king. The deshis transcend the skill of the aging master to preserve what has gone before.)

A lot has been written on the martial arts but very little on the science of pedagogy as it applies to the teaching of martial artists. For that matter there is considerable question as to whether art can be taught, as the best artists are often self-taught. This is true in the performing arts as well as the combat arts. Those men that I've known who bragged on the harshness of their master and the brutality of their training were invariably not too bright and were probably deserving of their treatment. From a higher perspective their physical skills weren't terribly impressive either. Together with John Porter, a ninja friend who taught me how to walk fire, I used to laugh about how some people thought that "mental discipline" could be taught by physical means. Like there might be a relationship between how many push-ups you could do and how well you could teach, fight, lead others, shoot a gun, or make a bomb. In statistics this would fall into the fallacy of comparing apples and oranges.

No great spiritual tradition that teaches single-minded pursuit of happiness leads to satisfaction, as personal desires multiply endlessly, forever creating new desires which create new dissatisfactions. Happiness is not a goal but a by-product of accomplishment and recognition of self-growth. Cherishing the growth of others, particularly those we love, exercises the larger capacities of our being and helps us be aware of our vulnerabilities. The call to teaching a way of creative development forces the learning of new skills while unfolding our finest qualities if we are taxed and fully stretched to the limits of our understanding. A real martial art has no rules and thus continually forces adaptation and creation through conflict. Teaching is a leadership behavior, and the relationship with the teacher is part of the modeling.

Since people do not generally regard wisdom, truth, or creativity as central to an intimate relationship or the mastery of self, they seek out relationships based primarily on biochemical reaction, companionship, or mutual self-interest. The same can be said for the selection of a martial art teacher. A true martial artist is concerned with saving your life. A master would also like for you to have one that is worth living, full of passion and excitement as you develop your deepest resources and finest qualities. This need not be rare in this day and age, as all the secret technologies of meditation, breath, and massage are widely available, and more and more knowledgeable students demand that their teachers exhibit the qualities associated with their credentials. This is not an abstract concept but a growing recognition that a teacher is real when actions are based not just on knowledge but the explicit presentation of one's own being through the personal experience of knowing. Knowing is doing. You must observe carefully.

For example, sometimes a martial system may be broken down into beneficial exercises and dances, breathing and meditation techniques, and combat and weapon applications so that all the knowledge is not in one place. If a country is conquered, the martial applications go underground. They may be hidden in what appear as folk dances or religious postures. The swords may be hammered into plowshares but the training continues. The Indian goddess Kala, a sexier, younger version of Kali, is often shown in the sword posture of *Dokko no Kamae*. I have learned many interesting techniques for strengthening my body through studying the movement of traditional dancers. The dancers of Bali have remarkable balance and control that appears full of life-preserving grace. The fighting application can be picked out of its aesthetic concealment long after the footwork goes from lunge to jeté.

When I met Kevin Millis the first time in Japan I could see he was a perfect vehicle. He had the build, diet, intensity, all the good ninja stuff. We became friends as he seemed to think I was wise and worth cultivating even though I was a lowly, old, and decrepit white belt in ninjutsu. I began to show this godlike black belt little ways to improve his already prodigious skills. He took my clues and covered ground in months that had taken me years to research. He has a very high IQ and learns fast. He would reciprocate by showing me how to improve my physical techniques. We had a great time teaching each other. (We still do.) Hatsumi would ask him, " Who is the teacher, Morris or Millis?" Our relationship doesn't follow typical hierarchical practice because we're Americans. A year or so after I showed him how to breathe and meditate properly, he could generate enough chi to show in his aura. When the grandmaster noticed his higher glow, Hatsumi promoted him again and then told him that everything they did from that point was a gift. He was a colleague by the rules of giri! Kevin had achieved the lesser enlightenment.

Kevin was horrified. No more learning hundreds of techniques with all kinds of toys. No more walking the dogs with the boss late at night in ancient Noda. He didn't want to be a colleague. He didn't know what to do. As far as he was concerned he was getting some chi. A little something extra in his ninjutsu! He was a California Boy. Surfing. Kicking butt. Lakers. Malibu and the pretty girls in the morning. Rock climbing in the off season. Spiritual stuff was pretty low in his hierarchy. He blamed me for spoiling his relationship with the boss. What if the boss quit teaching him ninjutsu and expected him to come around and discuss flower arranging, or levitate? His world had come unglued. He wanted no cracks in his cosmic egg. He was an urban, modern, American warrior.

So he went out into the Buddhist temple park in the center of Noda City where the roads come together. He went into the garden that has the little pool. He pushed all his energy down into his feet. Then he pushed as much of it into the ground as he could without dying. He stepped away from the spot. A desperate act of devotion on his part that struck me as lunacy when we discussed it after I discovered what he'd done.

51

We were roommates in the training bunkhouse rented from shihan Ishizuka's parents. I noticed Kevin wasn't getting out of bed after a couple of days and seemed to be real sick. Sleeping well into the day or catching up after hard night training was common behavior. We were whipped most of the time. Kevin looked like death eating a cracker, kind of dried out and definitely not himself. I said, "I can't believe you're sick, man. We hardly ever get sick." No jet lag, exhaustion, nothing. He looked like a sick puppy to me. He told me what he had done in the park. I couldn't believe it. I didn't know you could do that. He'd gone over to Hatsumi's to train after he'd fed the spirits of the place *(kami)*. Hatsumi told him, "You look like someone who has lost your way."

I loaded him back up after he'd suffered enough to remember what it's like not to have chi. Like many flower children, Kevin's short-term memory leaves something to be desired. Never ask him to remember anything abstract for you unless it is music. As an exchange of chi does carry some emotional content or intention no matter how clean you try to run it, I'll bet his perceptions were a little weird for a while. After I thought he was OK I took a sample and ran it through me for a check. (Every now and then I get this urge to surf.) He went back across Noda to visit with Hatsumi. Hatsumi said, "I see you have found your self."

I'd love to know what Hatsumi thought was going on. I don't know how he feels about experimentation on human subjects. Kevin told me a year or so later that Hatsumi had put a bug in him that seemed to flush out the meridians. The Indians, Buddhists, and Taoists all have purification rites and techniques for purging the body of toxins, as do Jews, Christians, and Methodists. When I joined the Methodist Church as a child, my father and the elders put their hands on my head. I fell to the floor, fainted, and threw up from the blast of energy. Some fundamentalists might regard that as casting out a demon. It feels like electrocution to a little kid.

Ninjas seem to work off giri by showing each other a good time. I always know when I go out to train with Kevin he is going to blow my mind with whatever he has come up with since last we exchanged information. It's a great pleasure to watch him teach and move. He has incredible skills. I wonder how the big fish are responding to him now that he's got a yacht and diving licenses. Octopi are supposed to be smarter than hell. They're probably heading for Frisco. Kevin likes his sushi.

Shihan Ishizuka took Kevin and I out to a great Japanese restaurant with private rooms and an elderly traditionally trained *geisha* (a woman trained to fascinate and encourage men) to entertain us after I showed him the trick of seeing auras. She fed us and cleverly played games with us while we got blitzed and laughed ourselves silly and discussed dreams. Tetsuji Ishizuka (The Fists of Iron) wants to establish a training camp in the coastal fjords and wilds of the resort mountains for the old boat and pirate techniques. Now that could be fun. A little luxury in beautiful terrain and then storm the yardarms. Let's try your *bokken* (hard wooden practice sword) on a deck that moves beyond your control. Traditional and modern assault courses with famous teachers, nets, and intersecting water slides. Wow!

I like to party with my student/friends. We pick each other's minds and verify our experience. At some point in their training they get to work on my house or lawn and plant something in the garden. I've had the football players moving furniture. There are always little projects that require more hands. Steven helped me with the plumbing. Randy and Steven helped hang wallpaper. Courtney's wisteria bloomed lavender this year. We call it sempai duty.

I'm told Hatsumi's shihans get together and attempt to dust his library once a year. Theirs is a Herculean task. I've seen his books. The shelves are full, so it's floor to ceiling stacks. He has a huge collection of more than three thousand museum-quality swords in storage. It's difficult to keep a heritage alive when you have limited living space as in Japan.

Many of the people who have studied ninjutsu have written about their experiences with minimal comprehension of what was actually being shown them. People come and go and take what they can use. Others stick it out, working their way up through the ranks, following their desire. Some learn the meaning of giri and amae. Some find their dream can be a nightmare. The ninja develops his or her endurance through external or internal energy. The end result is the same but the collection of experience can be very different. Ten can also be zero. People do very strange things and consider themselves martial artists.

I once read a martial arts book by some poor silly bastard who went around attacking martial art masters to see if they were really that tough. He got slugged by quite a few and could describe their techniques when surprised. He finally jumped some old Chinese doctor and herbalist who had an international but low-key reputation for chi kung and martial expertise. The boob woke up in a hospital dying of severe bioelectrical malfunctions that Western medicine couldn't explain or adjust. He had to hire the Chinese doctor he had assaulted to consult on his case. The old gentleman kindly saved his life. This young thug retired ignominiously from his stupid hobby after experiencing the real thing. He's lucky the Chinese like gamblers and consider fools touched by God. I would have handed him his first book and said "Save Yourself."

In most traditional systems, visiting with the *grandmaster* (the absolute head/founder/lineal successor of the founder) is equivalent to addressing the Pope or the Dalai Lama. Talking to Hatsumi is sometimes like hanging out with your eccentric neighbor. We had a couple of minutes to talk at the 1989 New Jersey Tai Kai (annual training party with the grandmaster) and Hatsumi asked what I was picking up. I told him that I was having a good time watching and learning from him, as it was a pleasure to know he was still alive. He laughed and put his arm around me and said, "I like to watch and learn from you, too." I don't think he was admiring my sloppy taijutsu. I haven't the faintest. I was beating the snot out of some great looking girl who had trained in Isshinryu and liked to wrestle. The girl and I were having a hilarious time. She thought she was dangerous. He said, "The next time I see you. You'll take the sword test." Then he said to my horror, "When the godan demonstrate, I'd like you to do something." I was a sandan in ninjutsu on that occasion. He's merciless. I'm going to have to properly learn the Kihon Hoppo.

A few moments later while I was in front of the crowd doing a cane throw I've done hundreds of times, my right arm went up instead of the left. My partner, *gokyu* (fifth green) Mark Kenworthy (shodan now and semi-retired as he pursues a career in organ music), started doing things we hadn't rehearsed. He got into his part. He started slugging me from behind. The whole thing got very spontaneous. It ended with me throttling Mark with the crook of the cane while throwing him to the ground after disarming him with a buss on the cheek. He thrashed in disgust admirably. The crowd loved it. We stood and bowed to the audience, then turned and bowed to Hatsumi and the shihans and skedaddled stage left.

He likes to test you. He can attack from a distance. It is the combat application of *Therapeutic Touch* (discussed in the Healing chapter). Kevin Millis comes over later and tells me I'm supposed to bow to Hatsumi first. He was embarrassed that his student was uncouth. No one has ever told me what goes into each particular grade, any protocol, or how to act at a ninja demo. The boss didn't seem offended. We were all having a good time.

Shihan Toshiro Nagato (former All Japan heavyweight champion in kickboxing as well as judo) asked if I wanted to be ranked in ninjutsu at the Los Angeles Tai Kai in 1988. Nagato went to Ohio State and can be quite fluent. He's very big, smart, and gentle. I'd been doing ninjutsu as a white belt for about six years without a promotion and thought of it as a hobby. I like the people who are in it, some better than others. It's a wild mix of people from all sorts of backgrounds. My progress always surprises me as I have no idea what I'm doing. I just trust my guts and pay attention. Like Woody Allen, I keep "showing up" at seminars of teachers I respect. Nagato-san told me to send Hatsumi a video of what I thought were my best teaching strategies. I sent back edited clips of some of the other masters I train with; I put in the beautiful girls from Hillsdale College's hoshinjutsu class dodging *shinai* strikes from the rear while wearing their white belts as blindfolds in front of a cheering crowd of martial art enthusiasts; I showed Ethiopian Toffesse Alemu defeating my best Errol Flynn imitation with Japanese sword and chain techniques; I showed him one of Hoshin's combination firewalk, beer bust and weenie roasts; I showed him my son Shawn, the power lifter, training with me with *hanbo* (three-foot staff) in a wooded clearing. After we were done beating and throwing each other Shawn delivered a little lecture on Vietnamese kung fu and the expansion and closure of the rib gates while breathing, then we meditated next to a wild rose. Hatsumi sent me a black belt through Kevin and a license through Van Donk. I wear it proudly. I like it better than my red and white belt, and even wear it sometimes when I'm teaching hoshin.

I've missed a lot of the traditional training as a hobbyist. I have been lucky in having very bright students who speak my language and had little preconceptions and no bad habits concerning the martial arts, so they approached their training with open minds. I will probably never again have so much fun as when testing hoshinjutsu (our smaller American system) against the ninja and discovering whether we could blaze the same path but as hobbyists. Yondan (fourth dan) from Hatsumi probably has to do with pushing through and keeping going when you're under psychic attack, as he promoted me after the demo and he was definitely jerking my chain as well as egging Mark on. It forced me to alter my programming in a hurry.

Esoteric aspects of ninpo that I have noticed include covert use of healing techniques by some of the higher-level players; telepathic exchanges—through touch, over short distances, and over vast distances; cloaking of movement; and great strategies for driving away the unsuitables. I will discuss how some of these are done, but if you want to be consistent in your practice you will have to develop chi. A teacher can pass that to you through contact as in the case of Takamatsu training Hatsumi. Or you can learn to develop your own way of achieving enlightenment, of becoming a *tatsujin* (indescribably harmonious spirit) through meditation.

Chapter Five

Meditations for Becoming Enlightened

Most people who purport to teach meditation don't realize the importance of some aspects of the practice and how it affects the brain. Meditation is the key to becoming a complete spirit, an integrated person, a whole human being, enlightened. The biological process of enlightenment involves encouraging the endocrine system to awaken the hypothalamus and cerebellum. These are the oldest parts of the brain and could be said to represent our deepest nature. They are concerned with movement, balance, protection, and music. They would also seem to be the seat of problem-solving, vision, and creativity if the cortex is primarily memory storage and word processing.

In recent years a great deal of research has been done on the effects of meditation. If you are interested in listening to a group of Western psychologists and scientists report to their colleagues, Insight Recordings has a six-tape collection of presentations from the Inner Science Conference for a very reasonable price. Write them at P.O. Box 546, San Jacinto, CA 92383. One of the points these researchers make time and time again is that meditation is hard work. The techniques I share here are empirically researched and provide useful shortcuts to avoiding entrapment by some of the darker emotional states or levels of awareness that can be useful for survival but aren't terribly helpful when you are taking care of everyday business.

If you have not mastered the simple techniques of basic meditation, you haven't a prayer of attaining your goal of becoming a complete human being or tatsujin. *Tat* refers to the void and *sujin* could be a water spirit. It does not matter what your religious background is, or for that matter whether you are religious at all, as the practice of meditation can deepen beliefs or eradicate them depending on the individual. Hatsumi recommends Americans attend the church of their choice. Religion is concerned with worship; this process is concerned with becoming. They are very different. What is important is learning how to discipline your mind and body so that energy may flow through you in the most beneficially natural as well as efficient manner. Meditation or mindfulness should become so natural to you that you don't have to close your eyes but can drive your car, walk about, make love, or win a fight without breaking your concentration or composure. Eventually you'll attain *mushin* (divine emptiness/innocence/absorption by the void) if you make this walk your everyday walk.

I will now present for you a method based on the ancient Tien Tao Chi Kung practices that are hidden within Bujinkan Taijutsu. All of this works and it all works together. You leave out any part, then shame on you. I'll emphasize the important secrets that are usually left out (or only passed on through oral tradition). There are worse penalties than boredom for doing this wrong, so read this over and approach the subject with caution and pure intention. If you're careful and maintain the right attitude by using the Secret Smile, you can have a lot of fun. Practice is more important than intensity or sincerity.

The essential aspect of meditation is relaxation. Medical researchers refer to this as the relaxation response. In the first phase the relaxation response is elicited to open the door for change; the second phase is used to reprogram or rewire the mind with fresh information along desired lines; the third phase is exploring the subconscious, group consciousness, and the process of melting away dualism. Let us remember there is no mind-body dichotomy so what you do affects all. Each individual's experience of certain techniques will be different but the principle remains the same. For example, where my inner vision is relaxed and filled with interesting challenges, my friend Mike Cornelius is constantly doing battle as he learns about his inner rage and competitive nature. Another friend who is enamored of Aleister Crowley suffers enormously for every piece of the inner puzzle gained. Entering the inner world of consciousness is a lot like playing Dungeons and Dragons. Many ancient cultures devised alchemical recipes and visionary exercises for improving oneself. All include meditation, but often only the outer forms or postures are preserved or understood by those unwilling to dig a little deeper or go behind the facade.

"The Lord loveth an upright man" is a true statement and on one level has to do with posture or keeping the back straight as possible. This is very difficult for the neophyte who probably doesn't have much sense of inner balance and doesn't yet have the confidence to allow his bones to support his muscles so he can move freely from his axis. If you've trained in ninjutsu or some schools of kung fu you'll notice there is considerable emphasis on keeping the back straight and the bones aligned in most of the movements. The postures for sitting in meditation are designed to provide a stable base for the beginning meditator and nothing more until he or she develops their chi through the training of the breath. Sitting up straight is what is important. Occultists refer to this as developing the spiritual body; Togakure Ryu ninjas describe the back straightening process as following or being lifted by an inner light, similar to an esoteric Christian description. The importance of the spine in spiritual doctrine is even reflected in the Latin names of the bones—foramen magnum (Mouth of God) and sacrum (Vessel of the Sacred). Translation of corresponding Chinese acupuncture points in Taoist scrolls renders Heaven's Seat and Seat of the Ocean. The burning sword of Tibet and the sword surrounded by a fiery dragon are both symbols for the spine, as is the serpent-entwined staff of the Greek caduceus of healers and the serpent in the tree for those who work with the living. So much for an esoteric excursion into universal visionary symbology. Here's the first lesson, which is to prepare the body.

Sit in a chair so that your knees are beneath your hips. Pull your shoulders back and then down so they are centered below your ears and your ribs are forward. Tuck your chin in slightly as you tilt up the back of your neck and head as if you were being lifted by your ears or imitating an elf. Close your eyes and pay attention to the back of your eyelids. Raise your tongue so it presses lightly against the roof of your mouth, the touching point above your upper two front teeth. (If you wear dental apparatus that keeps this from happening, forget vanity and get rid of it while you meditate.) This seal of the mouth is critical and one of the secrets passed in oral tradition. If you don't do this you risk severe damage to your brain stem and exquisite pain. Let your hands drop together in your lap in whatever manner they fall comfortably. Notice how this naturally straightens your spine and is not particularly uncomfortable if you have any strength in your lower back at all. If your lower back is weak, you may have to lean against a wall or tree and use pillows until you get it right. Edgar Cayce, the famous sleeping seer, was fond of pine trees. When you do get it right, you'll know because you'll be able to hold the posture for a long time without strain.

It's balance not muscle that allows the skilled meditator to hold a posture for long periods of time. In fact, some research indicates that meditation does not contribute to relaxation as much as balance and internal harmony. You may find the attentions of a chiropractor or massage therapist of some value in the beginning stages, and if you're a martial artist you'll enjoy their skills for more mundane reasons. Meditation that is done lying down is worthless for achieving the kundalini but can be useful for practice in deepening relaxation, visualization, and healing. (Dr. Rammamurti S. Mishras, *The Textbook of Yoga Psychology.* New York: The Julian Press, 1963.)

Energy moves through tight muscles slowly, so trying to meditate through strain is largely a waste of time. Sitting in a chair works; it was fine for Egyptian gods and Chinese faeries who valued stillness over contortion. For many Westerners the very stable lotus position which provides a seat will probably be too painful to derive its mystical benefits. A simpler seat used by the Japanese in both common and meditative practice is called *seiza* (sitting on one's heels, knees together to the front, ankles raised or lowered or held to the outside of the hips depending upon foot flexibility), with everything concerning the spine still applying. Another preferred seat of the mystic is called *fudosa* (the sage seat/the seat of powerful compassion/wind way meditation posture), and I've seen most ninjas alternating between it and seiza for meditation and simple observation. Some martial artists belittle the sage seat as they are not flexible enough to move out of it with ease, but with a little practice you'll be surprised to find that it's no impediment to fast action. The *samurai* (military ruling class that served the tyrant shoguns until corrupted by mercantilism) liked it a lot.

The sage seat is best accomplished by crossing the legs like the proverbial red Indian chief while seated on a *zafu* (small, round, pillow or hard pad that raises the hips above the knees). One heel is tucked under to press against the perineum while the other foot is turned to rest against the tucked leg's shin. The perineum press is important, particularly when working on your sitting smile.

Once you have mastered sitting in an erect and still position with your bones balanced so your muscles can just hang relaxed, you can begin working with the breath. Being still allows you to feel subtle differences in your body as you experiment with developing your ability to efficiently process oxygen to ignite the blood. Chi kung breathing uses a simpler formula than many of the yogic techniques but the end result is the same. Your breathing should be slow, silent, and seamless.

Seamless means there is no catch; the transition from inhale to exhale is so smooth that an observer cannot tell if you are breathing in or out when watching your shoulders or upper chest. As you breathe in through the nose, you allow your sinuses to fill as you press outward and downward with your stomach and groin muscles in a relaxed manner, allowing your lungs to completely fill with air. This is going two steps below diaphragmatic breathing as practiced by musicians and singers. With a little gentle persuasion the ribs at the front and back can also be expanded to bring in even more air. After all, you are going to need to run in an extremely efficient manner considering your goals. Breathing this way feels a bit like a cobra spreading its mantle, which is another common symbol in the martial arts. Air is our most easily attainable source of food and energy. No air, no Self, no life as we enjoy it.

Once you have made the relaxed, seamless, giant inhale a normal and easy part of your practice, add the following to your ever more complex but easy technique. As you exhale, slowly collapse your ribs and bring in your stomach muscles until it seems your very intestines are wrapping around your lower spine. If you are weak you can extend and exaggerate this tightening and loosening to include every muscle in your body with each breath, giving you the advantage of continual relaxed dynamic tension exercise. You may recall the description from the *Tao Te Ching* of the master who holds power yet doesn't seem to do anything. This practice is important on many levels even if it is not particularly dramatic, which also accounts for it not being well known. It is sometimes referred to as "the baby's breath" by Taoists as this is how the little tykes breathe; Hatsumi jokes about having very young energy and ninjutsu being a baby art. There is a beginner's body as well as a beginner's mind necessary for development on the Zen, Chen, or Tien path. It may not be pronounced the same but it's all the same nonetheless.

Now that you've discovered or rediscovered how to breathe for depth and power, you'll quickly find this method absorbs the high chest breathing you were doing before. Usually after a few hours of practice this becomes the way you breathe all the time, particularly if you remember to do it when you're walking or driving. If you're moving about it's not necessary to keep your eyes closed but all other references to relaxing, aligning the bones, and balancing on the spine still apply. It might encourage you in your studies of this type of breathing to know a 1987 survey of cardiac arrests at the Menninger Clinic (quoted with great regularity in Rodale Press's various publications) reported that all heart attack victims represented in that survey sample were high chest breathers. One hundred twenty-seven out of one hundred twenty-seven is a fairly conclusive little study. New drugs have been launched on far less evidence. High shallow breathing is also associated with paranoia and anxiety attacks as well as fainting. Learning how to breathe properly is critical to longevity as well as to quieting the mind.

When you've achieved four to six breaths a minute as normal you may want to experiment with faster inhalations and long slow exhalations. In deep meditation you may find a cycle of breath can take up to a minute. You may find that after a while you can also hold your breath for ridiculously long periods of time, which is useful when hiding or underwater or, if your chosen lifestyle is particularly hazardous, both. The morning is a good time to meditate. Before one goes to the dojo or kwoon, it's a good way to get settled even if you plan to meditate with your class later. The Togakure Ryu ninjas like to do it before performance or entering the territory of the opponent, rather like a prayer to enhance their chances of coming home to Mama. It's different from pumping up. Gatherers of intelligence try to avoid the way of cannon fodder.

One of the best times to meditate, in my opinion, is after sampling an anodyne you've learned to trust. The colorful sunset is fading after a two-day blizzard in January, and the wind chill is about twenty below as you face West and prepare to face the forces of night and death. Build a fire in the Franklin stove so you'll have warmth at your back. Put on some Carlos Nakai, an American Indian flautist and singer of singular power. This probably won't win me many sidekicks, but you should be sitting in fudosa or cross-legged like Chief Sitting Bull or Chief Red Cloud and prepared to do thirty minutes at least. The feeling is something like divine laughter for being crazy enough to participate in Inuit shamanism. It's a little like how a lifetime trainer in the martial arts feels. There's a certain "I'm still here!" about it which is part of the competency of doing it right, that's pumped by a hell of a rush as your animal survival mechanisms seek inner warmth. It's called "The Pleasure Principle."

I have a friend, Ed Purchis, a retired GM exec, who likes to go canoeing in the winter predawn, when it's quiet on the mid-Michigan lake and the water is coagulating from the cold. It's lonely as a leper's picnic. No one is out there sharing this magical if frigid moment with him. Even his wonderfully adventurous and curious wife, Kay, does not share this particular adventure. I liked it a lot, but it's a hard sell. The water actually grates as you slice through it, and the mist can be very odd.

After Kevin Millis and I had spent some time rooming together in Japan on one of Stephen Hayes' tours of historical sites important in ninja history, he suddenly asked me one sunny cold morning, "What the hell are you? You only take one or two breaths for every three or four the rest of us take and you smoke. You awaken instantly and know exactly where you are and where everyone else is. How do you do that?" He was an observant lad, even when freezing his ass off. I should have said, "I trust in God" but instead I said, "Oh, that's just chi kung. Even a child can do it. Let me show ya."

Quietening the mind is the quintessence of all the skills necessary for enlightenment. It is absolutely necessary to stop what we normally regard as thinking. As one of my early senseis told me, "You must think the thought which is not thought!" I worked on that little gem of a koan on and off for eight years during my diaspora from the martial arts for graduate study. It's a normal human urge to better oneself. But No-thought or Divine Emptiness is a pretty fucking alien concept for someone who is trying to earn a Ph.D. in the industrial Midwest, home of Motown, apple pie, motherhood, Alice Cooper, and Chevrolet, coming out of Penn State, the U.S. Army, small towns in the mountains of Pennsylvania, and the home of a Methodist minister and an elementary schoolteacher. I still love burning rubber. My shadow side is attracted to headbanging.

Fortunately, I was sitting in half-lotus one day on the sundeck of our condo contemplating my navel (which is a great joke on the operation of the *dan tien,* the spot two fingers below the navel which the Japanese call *hara,* and the medieval alchemists Seal of the Soul). My Puerto Rican neighbor who was working on his master's in business administration or some related subject at U of M, and who had put me onto Gurdjieff and Ouspensky wanders by and shows me Dr. Herbert Benson's little masterpiece on meditative research—his first book, called *The Relaxation Response* (Avon. 1967). (He has written better stuff since: *Your Maximum Mind*, Times Books, 1987.) In the first book there are perfectly clear descriptions of how to meditate from a medical and psychological perspective without having to misinterpret an archaic language or solve some madman's enigmatic riddle. What a gift. A guidebook on how to quiet and empty the mind for beginners. No *samadhi* or *samantabhadra* (total absorption in the object of meditation/pure intention), just silence. This I could handle. I knew how to shut up. This was science and I know the rules in that club.

The following is my interpretation of all you need to know concerning emptying the mind, with some extra challenges for the truly flexible yet exacting practitioner. In some circles this is called Dr. Death's Humbling Bad-Ass Brain Scrub. You should attempt to do this for at least twenty minutes every day, morning or night, until the condition of no mind chatter is normal and preferred. This is a phase one relaxation exercise. Phase Ones are to prepare the meditator's hardware. Everybody loves the Secret Smile (the most respected esoteric tool for transformation across cultures) as a Phase Two moving meditation. Most of the Phase Two exercises I'm using in my next book, or you can take the course or join the *ryu* (a stream/an integrated, codified, aware consciousness associated with winning under any circumstances/ fraternal-sororal-familial discipline that encourages risk and pain as a process for self-growth and development of leadership qualities for emergencies).

Start the brain scrub by simply counting to ten, one number as you inhale, one as you exhale. You are only allowed to think the numbers. Any extraneous thought such as my feet hurt or this is a stupid exercise sends you back to the beginning because all you are allowed to do is count your breath. Most people last about six seconds if they're honest, when they can't believe that second thought sneaked in and they start over. If counting presents too great a difficulty you might try going "ooonnnneee" with your exhale. This is called using a mantra, and any mellifluous sound will do while you are working on emptying the mind.

"Aum" is probably the most famous of all mantras and can serve the dual purpose of emptying and filling, as it means "All is one, both the beginning and the end." One of my students remarked, "Ah is the sound you make as you begin sex and Um is when you finish. Aum is another name for God when you are enlightened." This was without prompting and shows a remarkable parallel to the Tibetan translation of Jewel in the Lotus (om mane padme hum), which is a euphemistic pun for androgyny, as lingam (male principle/penis) is absorbed by yoni (female principle/vagina).

Or you can just make a loud humming or growling noise so your sinuses and skull bones vibrate. Make your noise as loud as you can and then begin to quiet your sound production until you can hear it only as a thought, and then keep turning down the sound of the thought like you're dialing down the radio until all you can hear is a high-pitched ringing noise which is sometimes referred to as the music of the spheres but in reality is just the sound of blood coursing through the round little blood vessels in your ears. Now that's quiet. When your mind is quiet like that you can hear a mouse fart, a useful skill when you are trying to detect the approach of an enemy or hear the admonitions of your true conscience. If you want to increase your hearing, pay attention to the root of your tongue and focus your listening as far from your body as your mind can easily remember. You may get a surprise.

The object is not to improve hearing, however, but to remove extraneous noise. You want a quiet, smooth-running brain that allows easy access to what is stored there. A Cadillac engine of the mind. You don't want a sleepy, moody, ignorant, slow, or jerky brain with a bad memory as a result of not knowing how to do basic preventative maintenance. It's time to change the oil! I'll bet you're still clinging to useful thoughts like $2 + 2 = 4$ even though you had the principles pat for years. How many jingles do you have stashed in there? Dinah Shore hasn't sung for me in such a long time yet I'll always see the U.S.A. with her out-flung arms blowing a kiss. If you can't turn it on and off, you don't control it—something else does. On one level it's the difference between external and intrinsic motivation; on another it's simply a matter of ownership and the normal human desire for quality, particularly when quality translates as having a more interesting and healthy life. Most people treat their most valuable possession like it was somebody else's unattractive dog.

Now once you've stilled the mind and made it quiet, observe how thoughts arise. As they do, just let them slip by without attaching or getting involved with them. Let it be, or let them go, or objectively observe as they float through your consciousness. Once you understand the mechanics of their movement, begin to trace the insectile thoughts with no interference beyond observation or attention without attachment. This exercise is sometimes referred to as The Witness. Once you have examined the contents of your ego or learned self, you can begin the process of debugging your software by simply not feeding unwanted thoughts. Purposively withdrawing your awareness keeps the thoughts quiescent and weak until they simply fade away. You dial them down, you still your mind. You turn off the radio. This is also a good process for dealing with addictions.

Another method which I have little faith in but offer anyway is "the gopher-whacking exercise," where one tries to push back each thought as it arises. This only leads to frustration and is usually given up if the initiate is taught the dialing-down or passive mind methodology. Beating up yourself strikes me as self-destructive regardless of what is being damaged. It's using a sledgehammer where an eraser provides a cleaner transition. If you're drawn to this manic kind of intensity read Crowley's *Magick: In Theory and Practice* (Dover, 1976). He offers some exercises for those who hate and fear their body which only a Victorian could see in a positive light.

After a month or so of mind-scrubbing you may notice that you're pretty hard to distract and your access to memory is fast and accurate with the exception of trivia, which takes a while because it is now properly categorized. People who never go through this process often spend their whole lives in pursuit of trivia, no pun on the game intended.

The result of this process is clarity of thought, often accompanied by much greater access to the subconscious—accomplishments that are hard to denigrate. It also has the additional benefit of greatly slowing the heart rate and sometimes lowering blood pressure. Research on meditators indicates they score significantly younger on tests of biological aging. The intestinal breathing greatly facilitates digestion and evacuation, which are also associated with longevity. The need for caloric intake often drops to about a thousand per day, which research in the last ten years strongly correlates with low disease incidence and longer life. There is a tendency to become more of a vegetarian in your selection of food and simultaneously to acquire a genuine liking for raw flesh. Takamatsu (thirty third grandmaster) decried modern cooking methods, many of which correlate with cancer, as being a source of weakness. There is a reason you feel energized after a snack of sushi or sashimi. Proper meditation increases your physical as well as mental efficiency. Not having to eat as much and being primarily vegetarian is a considerable advantage on a forced march or when traveling in hostile territory where a cooking fire could betray your presence. Do you need any other reasons why meditation might be useful to a warrior?

Now that you've emptied mind through passive reflection, the question becomes what do you want to put in there that might make your life more interesting? Meditation can increase analytical skills and memory and rejuvenate the endocrine hormonal systems, referred to by the ancients as chakras, as well as strengthen the parasympathetic systems which can be considered our immune system. The following are various ways to build the "inner light." The first is a kung fu exercise that is part of Taoist esoteric yoga and requires a little imagination on your part. You might record the instruction to play to yourself as you practice or have a friend read you the "recipe" while you are mastering the technique. Or buy the tape set that accompanies this book (available from Eurotechnical Research University's school of Polemikology basic and advanced meditation courses). We start Phase Two with the infamous Secret Smile.

First hit the proper meditative position that you like the most. Close your eyes and slow your breathing. Balance your spine in an upright position and put your tongue up. Put a smile on your face. At least lift your cheeks, so the corners of your mouth turn up if you no longer remember what a smile is. Tighten up your toes until they really hurt and then release them. Do this three times. Once the pain has stopped, pay attention to the relaxed feeling concurrent with it stopping and move that relaxed feeling from the sole of your foot to your ankles and then up to your calves. Bring it around your knees into the heavy muscles of the thighs and allow them to soften and relax. You may feel yourself settling into your seat as you allow the hips and pelvis to settle. Picture your thorax as a bowl or barrel (grail or vessel) filling up with relaxation. Let the intestines, stomach, and lower back fill up. Allow the relaxed feeling to flow up into your chest, upper back, and shoulders so that it overflows into your arms and down to your fingertips. Let your arms fill up until the relaxed feeling begins to move up the back of your head and around your neck, coming up over your ears and skull to rest behind your eyes. Catch the feeling with your relaxed tongue, mix it with your saliva, and swallow it down to the bottom of your belly, where you swirl it around.

Instead of emptying your mind, remember a time you did something you were not only proud of, but other people recognized your achievement. It doesn't matter what it was or how old you were. Pay attention to how you felt. Erase the people, event, and reward and keep the feeling. Take that feeling down to your feet and breathe it through your body following the same procedure you just did with the feeling of relaxation, but this time you don't have to tighten your toes. Bring it over your head, mix with the saliva, swallow, and allow it to mix with the relaxed feeling and then begin the cycle anew. Do this for three or more cycles of breath.

Picture a time when you were laughing so hard you literally fell down, cracked up, and totally lost it. Take out the joke or situation and hold onto that feeling of wild laughter and breathe that through your body, starting at your feet and ending in your belly. Mix it with the first two and breathe all three through the cycle.

Now, remember a time when you were in love and felt loving. Take out the loved one and the situation and hold onto that wonderful feeling. Take that down to your feet and bring it up through your body over your head, to swallow it down and mix with the other feelings. Then combine the four to breathe through your body following the identical procedure. The next segment is rated R and those under 18 must have the permission of their parents or guardians to continue.

If you're sexually active, remember the best orgasm you ever had, and if male, hold onto the moment just before ejaculation and breathe that feeling through your body (as you probably don't want to stain your trousers and the male orgasm is often too short for this exercise). If female, let it rip as you breathe that through your body from the tip of your toes to the top of your head, down behind the eyes, through the tongue, and back to the belly of the beast. This is the power behind the Secret Smile and one of those important little tantric items usually regarded as oral tradition. Once you've succeeded in combining all these feelings and moving them from your feet to your head and back to below your stomach, memorize the process. Make it part of your daily practice until it is so easy that it just becomes background sensation for any other exercise or a warm-up that sticks with you.

. The Secret Smile is a process for truly internalizing feelings. The feelings you have just internalized are also referred to as relaxed calm, confidence in your abilities, happiness, love, and ecstasy. You could say you're just making yourself cool, confident, happy, and sexy. I like to think of it as *Homo sapiens'* (Latin for what you is) natural state. With the distractions and turmoil of modern living it's difficult to remember that you once were and with a little effort still are in this state of youthful bliss. Zen practitioners call this remembering your Self. As your practice deepens, so will that concept.

Energy moves best through a happy camper and everybody

loves a lover. I taught a girl how to do this in about ten minutes a couple of years ago in California when I was out to train with Kevin and the look on her face was great afterwards, she was radiant. She said, "Wow! I didn't even know what smile meant." She couldn't wipe the grin off her face. I dare anybody to try to intellectually flog the mind into accomplishing that little exercise. Mental discipline has to do with attention, remembering, and creating, not how many pushups you can do on your knuckles. The Secret Smile also prepares the body and mind to accept as normal the movement of powerful emotions and sexual energy through it as a means for clearing and opening what Oriental medicine refers to as meridians. Let's move onto another exercise for developing "inner light."

Look away from the external light source. Close your eyes but pay attention to the phosphorous on the back of your eyelids. No color. Write down black in your diary of meditation events. (You are keeping a diary, aren't you? Don't you want to be able to explain to your grandchildren how you got so weird and funny?) Make note of any color or semblance of color you see. Hit the position of choice and, maintaining no expectation, empty your mind with your tongue resting against your lower teeth. Breathe like you used to and watch the back of your eyelids. When you're done with that, put your tongue up and begin chi kung breathing, continuing to pay attention to whatever happens on your eyelids. After you've exhausted those insights, begin the Secret Smile and observe throughout the five complete cycles of breath. Note any differences. Do this more than once. Look around back there; you may find some interesting surprises. If you do, they're yours. Scope 'em out, dude. It might be reasonable to check your progress this way at least once a week as part of your meditation practice. The little fat buddha called "Happy Ho Tai" represents this exercise.

Have you noticed that many of the legendary Japanese heroes are depicted as being more than just a little cross-eyed? I've a woodcut of Musashi, *katana* (mid-length war sword) held underhand, slicing arrows out of the air while looking backwards with his eyes crossed. Are we talking skill, art, or super-natural here?

Trevor Leggett (*Zen and the Ways,* Tuttle, 1987) tells us that the crossed eyes are an artistic device used by the Japanese to indicate that the individual was guided by looking inward or following an inner light. You might make the leap of faith from the picture to the godan test as representing something similar. If you've ever examined a Japanese pillow book you might have noticed that some of the positions are done with crossed eyes.

Meditations for Creativity

This next exercise from the Hoshinroshiryu is called Da Mo's Cave. Da Mo was the Hindu monk who traveled to China and, according to legend, revitalized the Shaolin Temple, introducing brain and marrow washing as well as chi kung and kung fu to the poor benighted priesthood of that far away and long ago era. Supposedly he sat in meditation in his cave for nine years. Like Christ, he felt it was important. He's usually painted with no eyelids, as legend has it he tore them off so he couldn't fall asleep when meditating. He's also the patron saint of tea drinkers. He's usually pictured as a rough-looking bearded gentleman. He is also regarded as the founder of Zen and sometimes referred to as the Bodhidharma, Da Mo, or Daruma. My first gift from Hatsumi was a watercolor of Da Mo. Hatsumi paints him as shame-faced and worried-looking with a flaming aura.

This exercise is designed to increase your ability to visualize and fantasize, and to provide alternative ways to access your subconscious and chakra system. If you're print and auditory oriented like me, you may have to have someone read this to you while you meditate. Most of the TV generation have no difficulty with this at all, as it is just like going to the movies. I don't visualize nearly as well as my students. What I do to remember and create is like what you do when you read a good author whose words allow you to sort of see and feel the situation he or she is describing. (Very rarely do I get the detail that the youngsters get. Most often my visions look like holographs. If yours work out that way, don't worry. It's all processed in the brain eventually. I'm told that us lower-IQ types have greater problems visualizing.) Just treat it like a story except that you are the main character and get to fill in the details as you want them to be. This exercise is definitely part of the oral tradition and similar to shamanistic journeying.

Hit the position of choice, do the PG-rated version of the Secret Smile, and then once you are relaxed and happy, picture yourself emerging from the water on a beach and then walking across a plain toward a mountain. As you walk along it seems as if your feet draw energy from the ground and every step makes you feel strong and confident. As you begin to climb the mountain you see ahead an old abandoned temple and graveyard, which you skirt but notice that there are bathing pools that still hold water within the ruined interior. You continue to climb and it is getting tougher. As you begin to tire and lean against the rocks and trees, you find that you can draw strength with your hands as well as your feet, and that gives you more energy to continue your climb. Ahead of you on a slightly different trail you see a cave with an inviting entrance. You go toward it and a guardian wearing a cloak that masks identity gestures to you to enter and bows so you feel accepted and a bit like a well-loved king or queen.

You enter the cave and find a long, downward-descending tunnel with phosphorescent walls that glow with enough light to see. This descending ramp opens into a large subterranean room. In the back at quite a distance there is a bed of glowing lava. On your left is a tall podium supporting a large leather-bound tome which has written across it in words of flaming gold, "All Knowledge Is Power. Seeking Truth, First Look Ye Here!" Behind this large book's podium is a room containing a massive communication and computer set-up, looking somewhat like the bridge of the Starship *Enterprise*. You can see three seats in there. One is yours. There is a young woman and a young man working in the room. They don't see you yet.

To the right is a great stairway with five steps. Each step is a different-colored wide slab with a doorway opening off of it. The first step is red and its door is heavy and barred but you can see that it opens into a rugged and ancient desert, and in the distance you can make out a city built from stone. The next step is orange and its doorway is a Dutch door looking out on a babbling stream that flows down through a forest to a vast lake or ocean. There is a ship approaching. The next step up is bright yellow and its door is intricately carved and looks out on a city that is both modern and ancient and seems to be sheltering many different kinds of people. Some even look like elves. As you focus your attention there, you hear faint laughter and music and the clink of glassware. The next step up is green and seems to be opening into the sky. You can see a bird floating. It's like looking up to an upstairs window. The sky is cloudless and light blue. The last step is tilted and spirals off into the distance in various shades of blue and violet fading into white. It almost seems to penetrate the dark rock of the cave in the distance. It is rather strange.

In the center, before you, is a series of rooms that are your living quarters. There is your bath, sleeping quarters, garden, library, laboratory, personal dojo and instructor, machine shop, stables, and kitchen. You explore to make certain all is as you want it. You are surprised to find an animal in a back room that regards you as its master. In one of the rooms you find a secret panel and in another there is a hidden trapdoor under a rug. You do not enter these at this time as they are dark. When you have familiarized yourself with the contents of your cave and feel certain you can return whenever you wish to improve it, for instruction or to play, allow your eyes to open.

My cave was initially rather austere. For a long time my bed was rock and I kept warm with the skins and blankets made from what I could capture. One day I asked one of my Hillsdale College students what her cave was like and she said, "I love my waterbed and masseuse. It's so nice to walk out into the desert with music blaring from the outside speakers when I want to be by myself." Angie Damm got me thinking that the cave might be wildly different from person to person depending on their interests and creativity. Da Mo's Cave has a lot of possibility.

Blake Poindexter's empire of the South would make Donald

Trump green with envy, and Mark Robinson's has cartoons living in his. What you may find out the doors, behind the panels, and down the traps is part of our oral tradition, but keep in mind Togakure means "hidden door" and one of the Taoist schools is "mysterious portal." Be careful as you explore the surrounding domains, and don't jump out the green door. It's a long way to the bottom of the abyss. There's climbing gear in the war room or you might try to ride the bird.

You should explore Da Mo's cave as an exercise in imagination. How real and yet how crazy can you get? Because the mythos of the cave is based on cross-cultural archetypes, as your chi builds your cave will change and you may find some very interesting connections to exterior reality as you also discover interior deities. Kevin Brown would write the answers to probable test questions in his cave's study and keep notes in the memory tome. If something slipped his mind during a test, he'd close his eyes, run into the cave, and get the answer. He carried a four-point average in Physics. Medical students may want to use the lab and visioning screens behind the book to explore their meridians or direct energy and other biological functions. Experiment—it's your cave and everything in it is also you. It gives you a fantasy arena to work out your psychosis. It's full of surprises.

My son once sat in on a session of my college class. As I was describing the stairs to my students, he decided to look in his tome. He told me the pages looked like Swiss cheese and then pointed out that I'd informed him once there were major holes in his knowledge that he should start repairing. He was a great kid and has become a remarkably good man and world-class chemist, of all things.

A variation of Da Mo's Cave taught to potential POWs by Air Force psychologists was building their dream houses in exact detail. The reports of prisoners in Vietnam claim this technique was extremely helpful in terms of enduring boredom, deprivation, and torture. It is recommended in this process that one even attempt to involve the senses of taste, touch, and smell while working on the inner vision.

Meditations for The Senses

Smell

Hit the position of choice. Empty your mind. Close your eyes and keep them closed. Pay attention to the tip of your nose, the rim of your nostrils. Breathe in gently and focus on the quality of the air. What do you feel and what do the feelings tell you? Lift your arms and take a whiff. Drop them and see if you can still pick up your aroma. What does it tell you, aside from your deodorant brand? Sift through your own body odors and breathe in deeply. What else can you smell in the room? Who else is with you? How far away are they and in what direction? Does their presence affect the air temperature as it passes your nostrils? Can you separate them out by sex? Is there a difference between cologne and perfume? Keeping your eyes shut, crawl around until you find a partner or one finds you. Do not speak. Do not touch. Sniff them out. See if you can remember who this is by their scent. Take a peek. Right or wrong? Wander around and try again. Analyze your progress.

Human beings don't depend too much on the sense of smell for information, as that particular nerve bundle is about the size of a needle. A dog's is about as big around as my finger and so discriminating canines can identify one drop of urine in a thousand gallons of water. When I was younger and hadn't hardened my nostrils by smoking for twenty years I could always tell if a lady was in heat and at quite a distance. Takamatsu is said to have joked about knowing the washerwomen were on his mountain when they were miles away. Since I was a preacher's kid and didn't know beans about sex, when I first noticed this I thought something was wrong with the women, and as they seemed to take their changing odor in stride then it was probably something wrong with me. I do recall I had the sense not to ask about it. It wasn't until I was out of the army that I realized the value of smell information. Because I was achievement-oriented, smoking kept away one very potent distraction. It's hard to get through school when you can fall in lust by simply following your nose. The nerves for the nose and the genitals grow from and connect with the same area of the brain. The nose knows. In experiments with women coeds, researchers found they could entrain a dorm of girls to go into menstruation at the same time using scent triggers. (It is discussed in most introductory psychology courses and certainly physical anthropology.)

You may want to experiment with various types of incense when you meditate. Some are supposed to be triggers to higher states of awareness, but most strike me as a way to cover the smell of a dirty room or a corpse putrefying. Smoke from a cooking fire carries for miles, and a cigarette can be smelled for hundreds of yards in three-tiered jungle. Wool smells different from cotton or synthetic textiles. Different locations have distinctive odors which are intensified if you're blindfolded. Scents get attached to memories at a very deep level and you should be aware of their associations. There is more going on with smell than meets the eye.

Touch

Stuff your ears with cotton. Suck on a eucalyptus cough drop or some other stinky product to block your sense of smell. Take off your shoes and socks. Close your eyes, or if you're really confident tie on a blindfold. Clear your mind. Feel what the air feels like around you. Notice how the air that is inside your clothing is warmer than the air outside your clothing. Move your hand away from your body and see if you can discriminate differences in air temperature from the floor to above your head. Feel your way over to a wall. Try to feel the difference a wall creates in the air before you walk against it. Put your hands out in front of you and try to find a friend. How close do you have to get before you feel them? Try not to touch, as you're searching for essence. Find them, back off, try again. What do your hands feel like as you do this?

Put your hands behind your back. Stick them in your *obi* (belt), or pockets. Lean forward and pay attention to how the air feels on your face. Close your eyes. Use your hands' memory and go

77

find a wall. Go slowly and carefully, as you are leading with that which greets others. Attempt to find a friend. Try to identify them by using your face. Take a guess. Wander around, try again. Feel any improvement.

Pay attention to your feet. Sink your consciousness down to the soles or Bubbling Springs and see what you can pick up from the floor or ground. We tend not to pay enough attention to messages of our feet, yet they have the longest nerves in the body connecting reflexology, shiatsu, and acupuncture sites that affect every major organ. What are the old hoofers telling you? Reach out and touch someone. Getting any messages? Aside from blatant erogenous zones, these are the most sensitive nerves in your body. What are they telling you? Walk around some more. Walking is the most important skill in the martial arts, the best form of exercise, and one of the easiest ways to stay in touch with your environment. It is associated with genius, and many great people have enjoyed the benefits of walking. I have seldom seen a ninja run. Learn to pick up stuff with your toes. Go barefoot as much as possible. Do some taijutsu. Try not to kill yourself.

Close your eyes and boogie around your own house and property at every chance. It's great for training balance and sensitivity as well as memory. If you have a lover it opens all sorts of possibilities for training as well as laughs.

Sight

Turn off the lights. Train in dim light. (Bars are usually dark. People attack you at night.) Walk around after dark. Get your night vision back. Eat more blueberries. Sit around in the dark and bullshit with your buddies. Make the night your friend. Guerrilla troops always own the night. Read in dim light. Palm your eyes for a minute or so whenever you think of it. Massage around your eyes at least twice a day. If your eyes are weak, try ginseng and see if they improve. Wear contacts rather than glasses. If you need glasses, try to wear them only for tasks that require them as they become a crutch. You don't have to be in 20/20 all the time. Our eyes are binocular and the corneas are supposed to be adjustable lenses. You ought to be able to consciously adjust them to various levels of light and focus. Wear eye shades as little as possible.

Sit down knee to knee with a friend or training partner in dim light. Empty your mind. Do the Secret Smile and stare into each other's eyes for a few minutes. Try not to blink much, and get your urge to giggle under control. You're supposed to be observing with no expectations. Without breaking your stare, shift your focus a few inches in front of this person's face. Shift your focus behind them as if you were looking through them. Shift back to the face. Shift to the area between the ears and shoulders. Shift to above the other's head. One person should then close his or her eyes and breathe deeply while the other goes through the same cycle of observation. Switch roles. Discuss what you observed, and share your observations with the other training dyads. Some of what you hear may surprise you.

Hearing

Put some music on the stereo. Hit the position. Close your eyes. Empty your mind. Pay attention to the back of your eyelids. Try to feel what the rhythm does inside your skull. What area of your brain responds? How does it affect the phosphorous behind the eyes? Try a different piece of music. Put on some baroque quartets. Try a little New Age. Break out the Beethoven; see what Mozart does. Try a Gregorian chant or plain song. Sample the Damn Yankees. Whitney Houston. Ravi Shankar. INXS. Enigma. What really lights you up? Run the Secret Smile to music. Try a subliminal tape. (It's useful to know when they're being used even if you can't do much about it. Keeps down the shoplifting. Increases the confession rate. Increases your chances of getting lucky. Builds your self-esteem. Speeds healing. Reduces vice.) Observe the differences. Figure out the benefits. You have to listen with your feelings as well as your ears.

According to legend, Pythagoras, the inventor of geometry and probability, spent years studying the occult effect of music and sound on the nervous systems of his students and friends. The results of his years at this work were mostly lost when the library at Alexandria was burned. In ancient times when there was no mass printing and all books were handwritten and rare, the burning of a library was a major catastrophe.

There are a few modern musicologists who are esoteric in their interests, and all agree we learn faster when listening to extended notes. Emotions are definitely stirred by music and some portions of the brain more than others. Some instruments and scales are considered very beneficial to meditation and are supposed to affect certain parts of the body as well as influence the chakras. Paul Abel, a local jazz musician, helped me try out some musical effects and wrote some very effective meditative music to support these exercises. Music soothes the savage breast (Willem Shaxpy, sixteenth-century English playwright) as well as entrains the neurological bioelectric systems of the brain. Sometimes when you don't like a piece of music, it has nothing to do with the music, but the associations and paths it stimulates. There's a lot of wonderful meditation music around now. (Hit the position to a Ravi Shankar raga and see what happens.) In the old days music was a privilege only royalty, the wealthy, talented, or professionally religious could enjoy. I suspect there are quantum differences between humming a mantra and wiring yourself into a modern CD sound system. I know there is, that's why I'm suggesting it.

Taste

Taste is a little difficult to work into a meditation unless you've developed the skills to move around in your relaxed altered state. As preparation for this exercise, attempt to hold onto the feelings from the other exercises as long as possible after each training session. Go to a really good restaurant that serves a wide and interesting menu, preferably of food you have never sampled. Ask the waiter's opinion in selection if you've no idea what is being offered. Make your order. Relax. Empty your mind of all expectations and concentrate your energies on your saliva, sense of smell, and tongue. Roll your tongue around your mouth and between your lips and teeth. If you are having a wine to cleanse your palate, inhale its bouquet, swish it around in your mouth, and pull a little air through it before swallowing. Pay attention to how it feels all the way down and note the aftertaste in your mouth.

Each morsel of food you put into your mouth, chew ever so slowly. Feel its texture as you chew and mash it about with your tongue. Smell it as it goes in your mouth and as you chew. See if you've the sensitivity to detect the living energy in the vegetables and flesh as you eat. Hatsumi says that Takamatsu could discriminate between teas grown on different sides of the same mountain, which would affect the moisture in the leaf. How does the energy of broccoli differ from a potato? Potatoes are cousins to deadly nightshade and their energy is easy to feel as they aren't that good for you, but we've adapted to them because they're plentiful and their inherent poisonous nature makes them easy to cultivate, as most insects and grubs aren't interested.

Sauces can be intriguing. Breads can have wildly different textures. What does the flavor and consistency of the meat tell you about the animal? I find wild meat much more interesting than the fare at the supermarket. Eating in this manner helps you to rediscover the sanctity of a meal as well as sharpens your sense of taste. On one level we are what we eat. Food comes after water and breath as a universal need. We tend to love who feeds and entertains us, thus the way to a man's heart is through bread and circuses. Awareness of subtle differences in taste, smell, and energy is a significant benefit when you are trying to avoid ptomaine or deliberate poisoning. How would you like the job of being the dictator's taster? Maybe you've treated the cook badly? The ninjas recommend shifting between blandness and variety and avoiding spices, as they stimulate the intestines and can conceal the beginnings of putrescence. This way's more fun.

Another even more fun way to train the tongue is in your kiss. Many subtle messages concerning health and degree of interest are passed in that junction. And you should take many samples to develop your expertise. Just ask Motown's Shirelles. Science need not be bookish or lonely.

Civilized living tends to deaden our abilities to interact with our environment as we become jaded. If we cannot have variety then we must pursue greater depth of experience to keep these evolutionary processes fresh and available. They are always present but are ignored, reduced, or forgotten. This is part of what the Zen roshi refer to when they say the process of enlightenment is self-remembering. Doing these exercises in the order that I'm suggesting will have immediate effect. This is the inner art of the life-giving sword, so fear no evil. If you want the outer art, go find a really good swordsman. I know a few who can stretch your imagination.

Meditations for Awakening Kundalini

Once you've mastered the above exercises you are ready to begin Taoist running of the microcosmic and macrocosmic orbits. Before you start this process, read the following books carefully and you won't get into any trouble like being possessed by a demon, delusions of grandeur, or epilepsy: *Awaken Healing Energy Through the Tao* by Mantak Chia (Aurora Press, 1983), *Qui Quong For Health* by Takahashi and Brown (Japan Publications, 1981), and *Zen Shiatsu* by Masanuga and Ohashi (Japan Publications, 1977). The ryus from which this information is drawn and synthesized are called Cosmic Fire Gourd, Golden Bell, Heaven's Way of Longevity, Da Mo's Cave, and The Immovable School Passed Down from the Gods. If you have accomplished the Secret Smile, made a friend of your body, and learned to value silence as well as accept your opposites—just do it!

Hit the position of choice. Breathe seamlessly through both nostrils at the same time while expanding and contracting your belly. Allow your mind to become completely still and empty. Look down inside yourself. Picture a ball of energy below your navel. Sink the ball behind and below your genitals. Pull it across your rectum. Tighten your rectum to push it up your spine. Hold the spine as erect as possible with the shoulders back and down, which lifts the front of the rib cage. As you inhale bring the energy up over your head. Be careful to keep your head slightly bowed with your chin tucked and your tongue against the roof of your mouth. As you exhale let the energy fall down the front of your body back to a point below your navel. Repeat with each cycle of breath for as long as you are able to sustain your sitting posture and state of no mind. If you cannot feel energy moving, just pretend that you can and imagine the process as I've described it. Do this every day, morning and night, for at least twenty minutes until you can feel the energy moving. Always begin your practice by running the Secret Smile. You want your body to be very happy; that way your hormonal system will cooperate and you will avoid paranoia.

Once you can feel the energy moving, picture balls of energy at the soles of your feet. As you inhale, draw that energy up to mix with the first ball at the base of your spine and draw it over your head. Your hands should lie together in your lap if you are sitting, or if standing, hold them in front of you as if you were hugging a tree with your elbows below your hands. As you exhale run the energy down to your fingers and feet. Experiment with moving the energy around and inside your body. Roll your eyes as you breathe and pay attention to what happens. Observe the colors behind the eyes. Whenever you get light shades of yellow, green, violet, blue, or white, attempt to increase their brightness.

Do not attempt to bring through an archetype, god, or spirit by imagining yourself to be on a particular wavelength or way of thinking and feeling. Sustain no-mind or what is referred to as mushin or Holy Emptiness, no expectations. Be certain your seat is very stable and comfortable. Pad your knees. You will go through long periods of stillness. After a period of days you may find that you sweat profusely. This means the body is purifying itself and removing toxins. When the sexual energy is drawn from the genitals, which may happen spontaneously, you may begin to shake as the orgasm mechanism is reversed and feeds energy into the body rather than out. In my opinion this is the oft-reported ecstasy/bliss and is strengthened and harmonized by the Secret Smile. Without the Secret Smile exercise it is more like thrashing and can be the precursor to the kundalini (serpent power/samadhi).

When you have finished a sitting session, get up and walk around. Give yourself a shiatsu massage starting at your feet and ending with knuckle knocking at the top of your head. Swirl your tongue around in your mouth and swallow your saliva. Give your ears a good rub and pull your lobes and haul the tops a bit as if you were the ghost of LBJ greeting a beagle. When you are not meditating, practice your martial art at least twice a week to keep the body supple. Walk at every opportunity. If energy levels seem painful, flick and shake your limbs as if you were shaking off water. Occasionally reverse the orbits and run the energy up the front of your body and down your spine and out your feet. If the urge hits you, run it in circles inside your chest and belly as if you were making an energy baby. Look down into yourself when you do this. It may be educational. Once again, maintain no-mind as much as possible and keep your tongue up as you do these exercises. You will thank me for this very important piece of advice.

This next technique is an advanced exercise I've named "Humbly Contemplating Your Navel." It is extremely beneficial to the art of cobra breathing and I wanted to include one completely original technique (not advanced by research) of my own invention so I could name it and perhaps restore some validity to a fine old tradition.

Sit in sage seat. Run your orbit. Drop your hands into your lap in the position Zen roshi refer to as The Mountain. Bend your body forward so if you opened your eyes you would be looking into your navel behind and beneath your thumbs. Breathe as deep and as slowly as you are capable, fully expanding and contracting every muscle in your body with each cycle of breath. Do this until it is painless and it feels as if your skin were breathing. Pay particular attention to the light show behind your eyes. Feed it energy and research what you see. Sit back up and notice how it affects your chi kung and ability to expand your lower rib cage in the erect posture. I recently saw old wooden carvings of men balled into this position in San Francisco's Chinatown, so I guess I'm reintroducing it. There is little new when considering the Ways.

The advanced technique is for the evening. Find a spot with rocks and shadows. Fold yourself into this position with your head resting on the ground before you and your hands completely hidden beneath your body but still with thumbs touching and fingers crossed. Allow your muscles to completely relax. Go into meditation. Become a rock. See if your training friends can find you. Hide and go seek for grown-ups can be educational. If you do it right you may get to meditate for quite a while! There are times when it is safer to be a rock than a mountain. Might be useful for a quick ambush, too.

Treat every direction up to this point as Gospel or at least like your mother's most delicious recipe that you don't dare change because whenever you do, the end product isn't what you expected and this is a very important bake-off. The ancient Taoists recommended you run the orbits as often as possible morning and night for up to ninety days if you want to risk the kundalini experience. Sun Tzu says that the long-lasting chi is best accomplished in the daylight of the hot and dry season, which is verified by my experience.

It is better not to bring the energy into the head until you've learned how to cool it. Some of the Chinese schools recommend just running the orbit to the heart chakra and dumping down the spine, not forcing entrance to the skull at all. I did not learn these safer techniques until after I'd had the kundalini experience. Some of my students have preferred these methods. They're slower, but safer. Once you have achieved the lesser kan and li, it's just a matter of setting aside the time to work on the higher techniques which connect *heaven* (the lotus chakra) with *earth* (the genitals). When things get weird, kick back, observe, and follow the light. It may well be that experiencing the kundalini is a result of doing it the risky way and bringing up the hot energy first. That way certainly forces you to learn how to use the energy if you don't want to be handicapped by burnt organs. A little caution, a stitch in time. If a little blue girl with a hatchet turns up, pay attention to her, but don't get off your seat. Good luck. God bless. Keep your tongue up.

Chapter Six

The Godan or Master's Test
for a Ninja

IN MOST MARTIAL art systems the black belt does not represent mastery but acceptance. Earning it means you have learned the basic physical skills necessary to be accepted as a peer or advanced student. It might be considered the equivalent of a high-school degree in mayhem. The second degree or *dan* usually means you can teach the basics; the third means you are a licensed teacher with some special skills; fourth is often concerned with dojo management as well as weapon esoterica, and in some systems it is considered the rank at which you are a fully certified teacher or supervised teacher directly under a master instructor.

The fifth degree means you are a master of the basic physical, mental, and spiritual fundamentals with your own contributions to make to the system. You have demonstrated mastery as well as contributed something unique to the system. In other words, you are not just imitating your teacher but have your own viewpoint. You have become an artist of the darker side of human nature in a socially acceptable context. It might be said you have awakened and tamed your shadow self. It must also be said that some masters' basics far exceed the norm in subtlety, effectiveness, and teaching skill.

Sixth degree *(rokudan)* and seventh *(shichidan* or *nanaedan,* for the very polite) are considered the equivalent of Ph.D.s or doctors and are usually referred to as "shi" or "shihan," which means head of school. These practitioners have developed chi, and are thought of as knights/scholars in Ninpo and Budo/Bugei. *Hanshi* or "respected master" is eighth dan or above in the traditional Japanese Budo. The title *Oshihan* is reserved for a master of higher energies or demon control who has not only developed his own source of regenerative chi (or creative spirit) but his students' students manifest. *SiGung* (grandfather) is the equivalent title in esoteric Chinese martial arts. In arts where spiritual training is part of the curriculum one will also have trained the intuition to separate right from wrong on a variety of levels. Not everyone will agree with this way of looking at martial ranks, but it's close enough for a generalist who considers his martial skills a hobby that has lasted for thirty-five years and resulted in eighteen different grades of black belt in five systems and three cultures with languages he doesn't speak or read.

The *godan* (fifth degree) test of Togakure Ryu Bujinkan Ninpo consists of the student kneeling in seiza with his or her eyes closed in meditation or terror, as the grandmaster, also in meditation, stands behind the student with a sword. When the grandmaster is ready he attempts to halve the student. It's the student's job to roll out of the way, avoiding the strike. To pass this test requires rudimentary skills in *telempathy* (feeling and reacting to emotions). From a mystical viewpoint, the student is accepted and protected by the *Bujin* (martial spirits such as *tengu* friendly to the Togakure Ryu). From my perspective, the student feels the sensei's mind change and avoids the strike, as feeling precedes thought. Because killing is not natural to the human being and must be thought about, this gives the student the minuscule advantage necessary to escape. From a Taoist perspective, the grandmaster and the student merge their spirits, and being in communion the student knows when to move. If approached from a purely physical perspective, the test indicates that your awareness has moved far enough out of your body that you can sense movement in another person's mind who is standing behind you prepared to strike. Concurrent with that sensitivity to the powers in your environment is a spinal flexibility so astute that one can be blown into a roll (or role when gathering intelligence) by the movement of the esoteric breath. All these perspectives are true to a greater or lesser extent depending on the student's perceptual abilities. In ninpo passing the sword test requires activating senses that are not normally used but held by all as part of our evolutionary heritage.

The grandmaster swings with his eyes shut, with the sword starting from above his head. The victim or person about to be promoted or dissected sits on his feet under the strike of the sword. Witnesses observe to ascertain there is no cheating, or to poke fun at each other's teaching results as Hatsumi, like justice, is blind. As it is no mystery in the ninja community, I'll describe my godan test at the Atlanta Tai Kai in 1990.

The godan test for a martial artist is the equivalent of the oral defense of a Doctoral candidate. It is the cumulation of six to twenty years of study. It's pass/fail and is over in seconds. As you can imagine, the tension is palpable. Picture, if you will, a small room packed with all the godan and above from the Western world plus the Japanese instructors and Masaaki Hatsumi. The energy from these individuals is potent. Now add in fifteen candidates for the degree whose anxiety certainly kicks up the level. Most of the men and women in this room were/are very powerful subtle energy generators. Trying to align yourself with a particular individual, even when it's the grandmaster, is not easy. You have to trust in him to really want to kill you, and in your ability to feel the *sakki* (killing intent). If the intent is not real, your protecting spirit will not emerge.

Hatsumi-*soke* (grandmaster) picked up a *shinai* (light bamboo practice sword), which is often used for this test in the West, as it is rude to kill a trusting but insensitive student. It is my understanding that Doron Navon, an Israeli and Feldenkrais practitioner, was the first and last Westerner to take this test with a live blade and one of two to pass on the first swing until 1990. He often serves as Hatsumi-soke's translator along with Rumiko Hayes. I was relieved to see this was a shinai belonging to Kevin Millis, one of the modern leather-wrapped ones that do even less damage than the traditional split-bamboo staves. Hatsumi-soke stepped in front of the table where his translators sat and said to the candidates, "As you do not get to train with me very often, I'll give you three chances to avoid the blow." Three strikes and you're out.

Dick Severence went first and set the standard for the day, as he easily avoided the cut and rolled away as the shinai hit the floor where a moment before he'd been sitting in meditation. Dick had been studying at least two years longer than I had and was in his sixties. Yondan to godan, so it went. Most of the aspirants avoided the strike on the first cut. A few took a blow or rolled too soon and were brought back to try again. My turn was approaching, my curiosity about to be answered. I'd wanted to do this for years. Could I as a hobbyist get on the wavelength of the preeminent martial artist of the world?

I crawled forward, sat on my heels in seiza, closed my eyes, and reached out with my feelings to connect. The first surprise came as I encountered "nobody home." Hatsumi was in mushin and I was in deep shit. As far as my body was concerned, no one was behind me. (There is more than one level of disappearing in this art and sometimes you don't connect things until you experience them. I had expected to be able to feel him.) I watched the white light behind my eyes and waited, saw a flicker in the phosphorous, and rolled. The sword smacked into the floor where I had been kneeling. Victory.

"Come back. No think," he said. I crawled back into position, another dream deferred! What to do? I knew I'd felt his intent but that must not be the object of this particular exercise. My mind went into overdrive as I contemplated my failure. Seven years down the tube. Oh well, what the hell! Compose yourself and see what happens.

Bam, the shinai cracks me in the skull. Strike two.

"You must not think," he says in English and mutters something in Japanese which Kevin Millis told me later was "These intellectuals always think too much." (Hatsumi-san is not totally without prejudice but he seems to direct it toward the things that matter.) At that moment I remembered Will Shepherd, who died rock climbing at night, describing his godan test as a feeling of great nausea in his stomach and not knowing whether to roll or throw up and then avoiding the strike with no conscious effort. I dropped my consciousness to the hara, or gut. My intestines were rolling, my body began to shake. I shut off mental process and waited, and waited, and waited. Suddenly I was on the other side of the cleared space in the room with no memory of the roll, leap, or crawl that allowed me to pass the test!

When the testing was over I gave Stephen Hayes a hug and thanked him for getting me involved in ninjutsu all those years ago. One of the young American godan who I'd befriended in the past approached me after the testing and told me that from his observation I had rolled at the correct moment the first time. I've given that some thought and explain my shortcoming in this manner. It is not enough to react to the killing thought. It is necessary to actually avoid the blow. In hoshin we operate from the thought, but the ninja responds to the deeper reality of the actual attack. One may be threatened but not attacked; responding to threat alone may reveal your skills to a subtle opponent and he or she could then use that knowledge against you.

In the godan test there is an exchange of subtle energy from the grandmaster to the initiate. The stronger spirit wins. That night when I checked my spirits in the mirror with sensei Sellers Smith and Dr. Mikey Fenster, there was a new face in the crowd. A white tengu! Transfer of chi is part of the equation. The sword test establishes and guarantees a link to the Bujin. If we think of this as a ritual of connection, protection, and healing, rather than escape and avoidance, it becomes an interesting example of hidden movements in ninpo. As I reacted to the feeling of the attack, I was missing the main event of being linked up; Hatsumi would feel that no energy went out from him. Viewed from this Taoist perspective, one should "joyously race to embrace the sword." However, one's taijutsu must remain good enough to avoid a live blade.

You are supposed to be a ninja whose fate often was to be unarmed against the sword. This level of flexibility and speed is greatly facilitated by integrating the mind and body so the spirit can emerge under the blade of the inquisitor.

On a political level Hatsumi may have been informing me that I shouldn't be such a smart-ass. After all, these other testees were real hardworking ninjas and I was/am only a hobbyist amateur with the unmitigated gall and temerity to keep coming back for more. On a deep physical level the hormonal drivers of chi are activated by the adrenals atop the kidneys (or less technically, by fear), and as a scientist and practitioner of chi kung and Taoist esoteric yoga I had figured out the "magick" and was treating it too lightly. Hatsumi was going to make me sit until he felt the proper amount of fear emanating from me. "This is not storefront tae kwan do takeyurdo, this is the thirty-fourth grandmaster of the Togakure Ryu lineage about to swing a stick at your head and you should pray to all you regard as holy that he misses. Now get with the program, as the blow is coming." Although I was sitting in seiza, the way my guts were churning and witnesses inform me my body was shaking, I think I was able to achieve a state of controlled terror and respect for the workings of universal reality and harmony. I let the cosmos decide.

I don't know what my body did to avoid his cut but I have seen poorer teachers' students slammed. I wouldn't go first unless I really had internalized the ability to feel intent. I've seen the shihan of all the branches and different races exchange that "Ughn! One of yours" look as well as celebrate skilled performance. We all know who we are. It's a very small club, particularly the Westerners.

I don't know if this is true or not, but I've been told that some of us have taken the test up to fourteen times before passing. It's considered rude to inquire but I know of at least two godan who are friends who said they paid and went through it six times. Considering the drain of energy, it would be a kindness and good etiquette besides to quit on the first failure, as some of the more respected ninpo players have done, rather than waste the Bujin's time. When Hatsumi gave the test at Tai Kai '92 in Atlanta the "strike-out count" was down to two. Two, you're out.

Out means go home and study for another year, as you are still a brick. Supposedly, in the old days with a live sword, when the Bujin rejected your test, you were just executed. Eight hundred years of civil war results in some novel tests of fidelity. Treat it like the real thing and you will get more out of it. Think of it as pass or die.

A blind roll out of a sitting position when you are meditating is not an easy thing to do if you have not lowered your center. It is especially difficult if you have hardened your muscles and made rigid and unbending your mind. It is easier if you are really relaxed and your body is flexible enough to follow your head. If Hatsumi invites you to take the test, he uses a shinai. If you ask him, he uses a *bokken* (hard oak practice sword). I preferred not to be concussed or reduced to taking it with a helmet to protect my wounds. Some of the failure stories are awful. I had waited three years for his invitation, and passing was second in significance only to going through the kundalini. It is both a great honor as well as a culmination of many years of preparation. But as they say on the boob box, "Don't try this at home!" It could be hazardous to your health. The test has nothing to do with hearing, and as far as that goes I tend to be a bit deaf like most middle-agers with a taste for rock and roll and automatic weapons in their youth. Some students attempt to pass by listening for the bamboo to creak since Hatsumi squeezes the shinai as he begins his strike. This counterfeit is easy to catch and embarrassing to see.

Now someone may ask what does dodging a sword out of meditation have to do with real-world fighting? The answer is speed, timing, and luck. We feel before we think. Feeling is the seat of the creative response, not the drilled response. Taijutsu will get you out of the way of the sword. Your spirit or chi will tell you when to use those abilities. If you're ever attacked by someone who seriously wants to kill you without harm to themselves, it won't be a face-to-face confrontation. These days he or she will hire some sort of filth willing to do that for money.

You get a lot of information through feeling someone's thoughts even if you can't read their minds. The intuitive range is quite great. With careful discrimination you can pick up speed traps and other fun consequences of living in this age. You find yourself next to the person you wanted to meet. You don't drive through the intersection just as the light changes as is your habit, and that is when a truck rumbles by, running the red. You bend over to adjust your shoe as a drunk hurls a bottle into the back of the chair where your head was resting a moment before.

Stories of near misses abound in Bujinkan. (I have often wondered if it would be considered a pass if the testee decided to go to a nice comfy bar instead.) Synchronicity is not to be sneezed at, like coincidence, as it is more like opening yourself to sustainable luck. Avoiding a killing strike could be described as loving your new acquaintance enough to fill the unforgiving moment with sixty seconds' distant run from the Victorian perspective of Kipling's perfidious Albion. The survival aspect that has the most power in the fight/flight syndrome has an "l." The godan test is a proof that you can enter the perceptions of your proto-consciousness and are now able to begin work on your true self. It is a beginning, not an end.

In a fight seen by an unskilled or biased observer, lucky, tricky, and sneaky may all describe the devastating maneuver executed humbly at the proper moment to do the most appropriate damage to an attacker. Now, that's a secret sword! It is almost impossible to teach unless you are an artist or can tolerate a great deal of experimentation on your students' part while preserving the core that is life-giving. Intuitive decisions can be superior to analytical decisions. "No think" does not mean stupid.

Passing the godan test in Togakure Ryu Bujinkan Ninpo indicates that you have reactivated your amyglia, hypothalamus, cerebellum, and brain stem, which are parts of the brain concerned with integration of knowledge, pleasure, music, and self-protection. They are the oldest parts of the brain and are sometimes denigrated as reptilian by misguided intellects who overvalue the efficiency of the cortex and fallible eyes. (The cortex may be little more than a memory bank.) When this reintegration begins to happen, your auric corona will run light blue. In some people it begins to manifest from their trapezius dorsi and hearts, somewhat resembling faint electric wings. In others this faint halo effect spreads from the neck and head like a hood. If the higher self is involved, the effect is something like a cobra. It would be wise to consider the myths and legends surrounding those able to develop the skills necessary to inner focus and interaction with such spirit.

This reactivation of the brain stem or becoming consciously aware of subtle input is referred to as the lesser kan and li in some esoteric systems of kung fu, as it is the stage of enlightenment attainable by all if they've the endurance or guts. It is why the *tengu* (demon spirits friendly to ninjas with the heads of birds and who once ruled in Egypt as well as Japan) refer to themselves as "only Tengu," realizing there are higher levels to reality beyond the *siddhi* of invincibility. The feeling of invulnerability will pass but is real and can be drawn upon when the threat is real. A real threat to a telempath is felt by the spine and seen by the eyes in the back of the head.

Often Hatsumi-soke promotes a Westerner for only developing one side of the equation, as he takes the long view. Sometimes the spirits speak through Hatsumi-soke and he shows great compassion to a student who really was not properly prepared by a knowledgeable teacher. I have seen some teachers actually invoke Bujin to intervene for the testee because their friend is/was putting on a very bad show for the other godan and above. One should subdue the ego and the flesh before this test. It is not necessary to pass it half-assed.

In the rush to embrace the sword, enthusiasm should not presage discretion, as the traditional test was with a real sword and the man administering it is still a certified channel. You will be remembered as an example of your teacher's skills if you are not self-taught. Hatsumi does not always move of his own volition. The last time I observed the godan test he asked for more strength to keep going when a testee was stupidly and repeatedly failing. Even his Japanese shihan never know what or who will move through him. A little paranoia is in order; some of the Bujin are malignant spirits appropriate to the horror of war. I have noticed the Japanese shihan both love and fear their soke. Study on this.

Chapter Seven

Portrait of the Artist
as a Grandmaster

"Just what is a martial artist, Master? How do I recognize a teacher of quality and goodness in these times of greed and false idols?"

The mission of the artist, regardless of the medium of expression, is to elevate his or her perceptions through study, practice, and intelligent insight to the highest attainable level within their capability and then communicate that knowledge or expression to their peers, and if teachers, to the wannabees. I believe there is a tenuous genetic component to art associated with intelligence. The problem that confronts all in the pursuit of original expression of creativity is the easy slide into mediocrity as a result of popular acceptance when one settles for the least common denominator.

In academics this can be seen in the ABD who enjoys the teaching but never finishes his or her dissertation and ends up in the junior ranks of professors, or is not granted tenure after four or five years of excellent teaching. In religion this is the con man who claims the calling and fakes the healing and establishes systems for adulation and worship rather than giving guidance from his own experience of becoming. In the martial arts this is represented by the shodan who teaches as if he or she were a master because in the eye of the public a black belt represents mastery, but in the eyes of traditional martial artists it's about the same as a Bar Mitzvah. Only godan and above are considered original thinkers with spiritual as well as technical expertise to offer. Hatsumi says, "Give the shihan the adulation they earn rather than the rank they've attained." The master martial artist is not just a gifted physical technician but has an additional role as a teacher and spiritual guide, which is seldom understood in the West or practiced in the East. *Sensei* means one who has gone before, and *shihan* means you finished the trip but have not necessarily reached your destination.

How many men in long-ago Florence understood what Dante was all about? How many in Poland understood Copernicus? Darwin and Huxley had to deal with near riots when they published their ideas in England. Hatsumi is regarded as an unidentified flying object in Japan. Good original work is seldom embraced by the more traditional masses until long after the pioneer is dead, with the exception of dance, novels, music, and maybe movies.

Now it has to be recognized that an artist in many ways resembles an outlaw. Just as the great writers and painters and poets (and inventors) must separate themselves from what has gone before to create the new, so must the artists lift themselves above their cultural milieu. Often that process requires extreme breaks from tradition or cracking the cosmic egg to see reality in new ways; seeing with a different perspective leads to different behavior. Where the outlaw destroys, the artist builds but the psychological root of the actions may be similar. Van Gogh assaulted our sense of shape and color. Monet, the effect of light. Wagner, our ideas of acceptable sound. Picasso, our ideas of form. Dali, our relation to imagination. Artists who are creative depart from the norm. The criminal, however, is usually not too bright and his destructive nature soon attracts the means of incarceration rather than liberty. The spiritual adventurer goes within and the terrain has both dangers and rewards, but to the outside observer little seems to be going on beyond someone just sitting around. It's not an easy sell. Those ideas associated with Crazy Wisdom and shamanism have so far made the most sense to me. The martial artist must not allow himself the gift of complacency regarding skill level when there are schools of clever people studying to beat the system.

Hatsumi remarks that the concept of martial artist is grossly misunderstood in America and probably in Canada and Europe as well. It's a problem involving a free-enterprise society that has industrialized its school systems to reflect a quantity-over-quality reward system; where someone can become wealthy by mass producing to fit the lowest common denominator or estimated taste. The destruction of the creative element starts in elementary school if the child comes from an enriched home. The child from a deprived environment soon comes to love school more than home. If children cannot rely on the teachers for useful information, they quickly turn to their peers. The public elementary school is where only the most intelligent and effective teachers—whose manner encourages a joy in learning—should serve, as that is when the child's brain is most hungry and learning most pleasant. We tend to waste it on pap.

In the martial arts, showiness often wins out over effectiveness in the short term. For example: You're proud of having a teacher who can show you how to do actual killing techniques in a fist fight. Do you realize what will happen to you if you actually murder or seriously injure someone? *Dim mak* is real; if your victim survives the initial onslaught he may find himself with serious handicaps unless he knows an acupuncturist. The highly skilled martial artist can drop you with a touch. The fist fight seldom goes beyond one punch. The good stuff all flows out of being attacked. Has he taught you how to conceal the body or hire an effective attorney? Are your meditation techniques disciplined enough to sustain you in prison where an athletic body can be the object of desire for many. No? Dumn. (I like spelling dumb this way, as being silent seldom equates with stupid in the gathering of intelligence. It is so much harder to learn when your mouth is moving.)

You're proud of having a teacher who is showing you how to aggressively move into proximity of another human being to exchange kicks and blows in a fight. Has he taught you that real human beings use weapons when they fight and treachery to win? That when you kick above the knee you will almost assuredly lose your genitals to a skilled opponent, and that most real fighters like a sneak attack and enjoy assaulting others from the rear, particularly when they are blinded by their own blood? Has he shown you some methods for dealing with multiple opponents, as many people only fight in groups, sport? No? Dumn.

Has he spent many hours teaching you how to be polite and fit into the company of strangers? How to safely avoid broken bottles, ashtrays, tire irons, chairs and other fun instruments of homicide available in most social situations? How about the avoidance and use of firearms and edged weapons? Has he shown you how to climb and move on various surfaces in free and cluttered conditions? No? Boring. You're spending most of your life on flat, smooth surfaces?

Does he somehow confuse the ruled elegance of sport with the brutal ugliness and chaos of battle when you carry no weapons and are far from home? Does he emphasize perfect repetition over practical utility? Does he enforce a lot of ritual that has no meaning to you? Can he explain down to minute detail how to execute the perfect fist, punch or kick? Are the movements powerful— and jerky? Are you paying this person to teach you how to save your life? Study on this!

A martial artist so thoroughly understands the basics of his tradition that he or she can depart from the expected and respond both creatively and effectively to the actual situation with the appropriate strategy that ensures winning. The enlightened martial artist has the further obligation to preserve life or release it as a sacrifice. His or her sensitivity should be so great that they can pull down the eyelids of their opponent as they lay their hands upon his face at full speed from a totally relaxed posture as a response to the opponent's chosen attack. Staged *kata* seldom seem to account for how bodies react when they're being torn apart, or for that matter, what the performer would really be doing if on the receiving end of serious aggression.

I've never seen a real fight last longer than seconds when one of the opponents was properly trained to accept and create a changing reality. A master or martial artist is not limited to one decisive strike but can escalate and control the situation by flowing with it and judiciously modifying their opponent's behavior through pain and imbalance. Such skill requires a deep understanding of all aspects of human behavior. Hostility and aggression prevent flow and slow learning. Humor and joy at being presented with an opportunity to teach on many levels is a characteristic of a mature martial artist. (I have seen the great practitioners break into laughter when giving a lesson in surprise tactics.) Fear paralyzes. A martial artist cannot fear his subject matter, however debased, or he will lose many opportunities for growth and practice. Study on this.

An artist studies form and beauty through his own experience of the world. A master artist is recognized by his own school as a teacher. A grandmaster is recognized by other schools as being able to teach their art. Hatsumi has been passed the shihan or head of school scrolls of at least nine famous Japanese schools to preserve. This is a ferocious undertaking. Within each of those schools are probably nine more traditions if the Buddhist liking for the number nine and esoteric numerology holds true, making Hatsumi the head of eighty-one disciplines. I understand he has taken some other scrolls out of kindness just to ensure the learning won't die. It is the equivalent of attaining nine earned Ph.D.s and a smattering of honoraries from extremely physical and cynical men. Inside of that he's a bone doctor, calligrapher, painter, actor, writer, fair vocal musician, magician, and only God knows what else. According to people I've talked to in Japan, he is considered in the top levels in each of these fields of endeavor outside ninpo, a Japanese Renaissance man. I know he astounds me.

Most good schools of the martial arts have their own etiquette, codes, belt knots, favored weapons, history, *kihon* (formal basics), breathing techniques, emergency medical techniques, and mental disciplines. In addition to the open techniques that are taught the public, there will be hidden techniques that are only shown the student after he or she commits to the system of instruction inherent to the school—unless he or she demonstrates their attainment prematurely. Usually every shown technique has a mirrored hidden technique as well as subtle helpers that may or may not be shared. I think these are referred to in Japanese as *ura* (hidden) and *omote* (shown publicly) but check into it yourself with a good teacher who speaks the language. It's a subtle area for investigation. Attainment of the hidden is always a rewarding adventure as it requires creativity, not just rote learning or repetition of what you are shown. Often the hidden techniques are not shared until the student achieves the rank of sandan in a traditional art—which accounts for the terrible combat and street record of some of the Korean systems based on Japanese ryus, where promotion by travel is of mythical proportion. Technicians tend to punish departure from the tried and true as taught to them. A combat martial artist studies war or life-preserving behaviors, not contests or games, so is always concerned in the ways of preserving peace. Artists aren't stupid and want to be allowed to do their thing.

I once heard Stephen Hayes say that Hatsumi thought Miyamoto Musashi, Japan's sword saint, had led a sad life. I'll tell you why it was sad. He was in at least three wars, the first one on the losing side. The losers are supposed to commit suicide because they were dumb enough to put all this to risk by following the wrong side, and nobody with any sense wants them around. It's a small chain of islands. There is no escape from the condemnation of your neighbor. Losers aren't supposed to contribute to the sperm pool. But he didn't commit *seppuku* (ritual suicide).

Musashi killed many master sword teachers in duels, which has grave karmic consequences in societies where skilled teachers are revered. He could find no student good enough to follow him as a master in his youth, and in his middle years they feared for their lives. He was chock full of useful combat information, if you want to live when your back's to the wall. For most of his life the average samurai thought it would be a great honor to kill him and at the same time establish their new school of the sword and famous reputation. He was *ronin* (a wave man). None would give him shelter in fear of the retribution and blood guilt they would be sheltering in their homes. He spent much of his teens living in the woods and sleeping in caves. He was observant, he learned from the animals. When he was thirteen he killed a teacher of the sword. In Buddhism it's a sin to harm a teacher. In his late teens he killed damn near a whole school when they demanded a group duel. Them against him in a big park near Kyoto. The samurai code allowed them to do this; they were all insulted. Musashi went early and hid above their line of sight in a tree on the highest ground. They being strategists also sought the high ground but felt safe in their numbers. He waited till night, then surprise attacked. Leaping down from the tree, he cut down the heads of the Yoshioka family school, one of whom was a mere child. He escaped in a running retreat through the darkening woods back to the city to supposedly end that bloodline and this particular feud.

He was an active, athletic man and stayed that way. He walked a lot. The duelist lifestyle leads to hasty travel. Musashi states in code that he was a student of Taoist breath techniques and had developed the third eye. He strongly recommended hiding combat skills in natural movement. One of the stories about him has him killing a tengu, which means he trained with ninjas. In his recently published fictional (but much loved in Japan) biography, the author has Musashi stating in middle age that he was fortunate to have never met an enlightened swordsman in his youth. For most of his life he didn't own much more than a sword. He raised a stepson, who may have died a hero, in a very haphazard manner. He never married though he did have a lover, whom he could not marry due to his miserable existence. The saddest part of his life was that he was a greater artist and strategist than swordsman. He was a fine sculptor of wood. His brush paintings are considered national treasures, and I've seen his cast sword guards in museum collections. He was an artist of enduring excellence and worthy of study. He died of old age around sixty after writing in one night a book on swordsmanship containing all he knew about it.

Most of *The Book Of Five Rings* is in code or very old language. Musashi exhorts his readers to consider the book as a spiritual guide, but most readers don't know how to read that way, as they are martial and military students. He did not get his skills overnight. He retired from accepting duels at fifty-five. Most people remember him as a duelist, but he was a great artist and friends with priests, geishas, and poets, particularly Takuan Soho. I don't think he cared a rip about what is commonly thought of as swordsmanship. After he was thirty-five he fought most of his duels with wooden training swords *(bokken)* or what was available when he was attacked. He killed the Emperor's sword teacher with a boat oar after spending the night at a geisha house. He called his way of fighting "two swords" as he had a secret one that came from the left. He was an upright man. He lived in a very bad time and had to educate himself with what was at hand. I like his book a lot. It is generally misunderstood by most readers as a text on winning swordsmanship rather than endurance, chi, and survival when you are the preferred target of many. It is full of traps for the unwary swordsman, as Musashi knew his enemy well.

A long time ago when we didn't have such professional means to distance us from who we were killing, being able to win a duel without incurring blood guilt was considered part of being a gentleman, but a master could completely change the attacker's mind. It takes a lot of time learning to flow under extreme stress if you haven't the heart or flexibility for it. You hate to give up clarity because some dirtball wants to fight. You are allowed to administer rude and abrupt lessons to the overly assertive if they attack or actually threaten you, as that is part of the way. Teaching the esoteric side of a martial art seldom pays well, as you're supposed to drive your students away, particularly if they seem inclined to abuse their power, or you can see that their heart is not in it and they would be better served elsewhere. This can be a creative process and a lot of fun. People usually will not pay to be abused if they are not learning. If they're smart you probably don't have to go full force more than once a night to illustrate a point. (You would like them to leave as friends if you've come to respect and love them, but you still must send them away. Sometimes it can be extremely painful to both parties, particularly if you have promised something you cannot deliver as they won't do the work to get it. Learning is two-way.)

If you're a ninja grandmaster you teach people different styles and disciplines within the styles, so they have to get to know each other if they want the hidden. You're supposed to lay false trails and ambushes for the unwary and yet keep their friendship. It can be like being trapped in a shaggy dog story. Rumors and politics abound in Togakure Ryu ninjutsu, but everyone is usually treated fairly or as they deserve, from my observations of Hatsumi. As we say in the sheltering mountains of Pennsylvania, "You give a fool enough rope and he will hang himself." A master of the dual mandala exhibits both sides at once. Many of the higher-level instructors have their own political agendas but cannot slip it to you in four ways.

An artist likes to personalize his lessons so that they will be fixed in the witness's very soul. The lessons become messengers to all those who would wish to see reality, which to an artist is creativity. The strategically creative consciousness state translated from Mikkyo Buddhism as the "mind and eye of god" never stops, it continually evolves. You're allowed to rest and make mistakes, but you have to keep going. Keep playing. It is not just the difference between the professional and the layman, but the lover and the slave, or the living and the dead. In tarot the hanged man is dancing. Hong Kong Phooey, the cartoon character for children, stereotypes with humor the life of a martial artist in America. It can become serious business at the drop of a hat but most of the time it can be your hobby. (Just your way of stretching and getting a first-rate, three-level workout. Things you don't use, you lose. A real martial art has utility in every aspect of your life. The United States needs more teachers of the heart.) Strategy has many faces.

A teacher of the art of enlightenment has the additional problem of being known by his or her students as well as his or her own actions, words, and deeds. Art requires human beings. Martial artistry is the stuff of legends. The students and their achieved levels are a reflection of one's skill as a teacher as well as the tradition

105

as a whole. The difficulty of the curriculum, the numbers engaged, and price are measures of popularity and appeal but the enlightened are mostly concerned with transformative power necessary for survival in all its variations. A college instructor has to accept who pays for the class. A graduate of Penn State does not have to play football. *A graduate of an enlightened ryu must manifest sentience above physical competence.* The competence is fun. One of the reasons Hatsumi could say with confidence a few years back, "I am the only true ninja in the world," was that he'd been visiting those who purport to teach authentic ninjutsu. You have to gather your own intelligence when your observers are naive. The ryus of invisibility hardly advertise. I usually don't put Skilled at Death Touch *(Dim Mak)* on my resumé when interviewing in the Midwest.

A *maharishi* (great sage/seer/teacher) is saddled with the additional burden of offering guidance and personal experience (wisdom) to the benighted if they ask and are willing to pay the price of truth. This is not trivial. The Togakure Ryu considers forty years of training—twenty for the yang and twenty for the yin—a normal course of study, with no guarantee you'll figure out the hidden. To learn all this stuff will take the rest of your life at whatever point you wish to enter. (Hong Kong Phooey worked as a janitor so he could study what he wanted, because he wanted to be good enough to be a teacher. The warning is clear.) You as a consumer have the additional problem of entering an evolving system.

I think it helps to have someone show you the basics. The greater the teacher's ability to transmit the traditional standards, the more you will enjoy and value your experience of the hidden, particularly if you have the open-hearted ability to treat people with respect, curiosity, and friendly reciprocity. The study of martial arts is a lot more fun than golf or tennis and has managed to be an embarrassing but absorbing interest of mine for more than thirty years. If you can avoid the sports and use the techies, you get to meet very intense and alive people, many of whom are compassionate and fun. In ninjutsu, like anthropology, they tend to be older as they've rejected the callow pursuits of their youth, usually after a long rough ride.

Quality in art is supposed to be transferable to any subject that interests the artist. Hatsumi's traditional watercolors, brush work, and calligraphy are as good as any I've ever seen. When he works in oils he tends to prefer the impressionistic and modern primitives. One of his oils featuring a huge golden spider with a naked woman in the web struck me as particularly perverse and funny considering his role in life. Many knowledgeable readers of Sun Tzu would pay a mint to put it on their wall, if they knew of its existence. It was in a Tokyo exhibit that I couldn't afford. The lives of Da Vinci and Cellini reveal diverse interests beyond the smearing of colors. Da Vinci's secret journals reveal a grave robber studying anatomy, and both he and Michelangelo were military advisors. Cellini was a swordsman as well as a sculptor and the only man to escape from the Pope's jail twice.

The Zen concepts of art include the possibility of the perfected movement that exists for the moment and then disappears, known only to the doer. *Haiku* (short Japanese nature poems) attempt to capture the feeling of a particular moment. Ninpo is taught more by how a movement feels than how it looks, as each practitioner attempts to make the basics personal. Hatsumi says this concerning the basics of ninpo: "The ninja's role in society is to protect the good. . . . Technique is nothing; the kihon hoppo is for children, a first step. . . . Movement from the heart is hard to see and understand but everything." This statement applies to any activity where the intention is the attainment of quality.

An artist is involved in transformation, not replication, but must demonstrate competence. A martial artist is tested continually in ways other than success in the marketplace. Some never get to prove the efficacy of their study. One of my red belt (beginner after white) college students of Arab descent was attacked while studying in Spain. He dropped the attacker screaming to the floor by unbalancing him with a nerve center grip while delivering a mallet kick to his calf. He quickly strolled from the bar before anyone noticed what had happened in the men's room. His wealthy father who had wanted him to take up tennis as being more useful now supports his fall from acceptable sport. Another student, a sandan who teaches high school math, told me he pictures how the problem is done and focuses on the forehead of the recalcitrant student. Breathes it at him or her and watches in wonder as they suddenly seem to figure it out. Another sandan who is an actress shamanisticly becomes her character and draws the audience into the action through radiating intent. She's riveting to watch—American *kabuki*. When I taught at Penn State one of my prettier students was attacked by a fairly competent rapist according to his rap sheet. His black eye, broken elbow, and dislocated shoulder made him very easy for the police to identify. She didn't even get a bruise. Budo is not the same as publishing a fine novel, or being in the movies, but martial artistry in the realm of single and small group combat with a little spiritual development thrown in for the sensitive seems as good a way as any to get a life.

Art requires passionate interest in people, material, or action. Grace or harmony of movement appropriate to the situation is part of art and is supported by the laws governing self- defense. Those who follow the light do not fear the darker side of endeavor. Warriors understand conservation, hunting, and the necessity for pruning back the excessive. Enlightened warriors remember the Golden Rule and can mirror their attacker's intent, but that type of neurolinguistic programming fades before the art of transformation necessary to love your enemy and give him every opportunity to surrender while protecting your interests. It's more fun and keeps it challenging.

Pressing down on a bone-shattering wrist and shoulder lock is a comfortable position for skillfully negotiating with a barbarian. A well-applied ninja shoulder lock is the equivalent of religious conversion for many ruffians who thought they could fight and did not know how to fall. Praising your enemy's weakness can be a blessing in disguise.

Insincerity is another matter altogether. Every religious writer I have ever read seems to ignore that the searcher must build the connection to the Void with his or her own inner direction. I have yet to see it happen from the other direction. Paul Brunton gives an excellent exterior description of the Void or Sacred Emptiness in his book *The Secret Path*.

Hatsumi describes one of his colleagues in the Togakure Ryu as a man whose swordwork was so skilled that he witnessed him draw his sword and cut the wing from a bird in flight. Takamatsu, a man who could so terrify attackers that they would see death as attractive, did not give the scrolls to this incredibly skilled person. Think for a moment what it would take to clip a wing with *iado* (Japanese art of sword drawing) let alone sneak up on a bird. Balance, silence, speed, prediction, or timing as the wing must be open, familiarity with your weapon. All good left-brain, right-handed, masculine stuff. The right-brain, left-handed, feminine stuff regards this act of butchery from the viewpoint of, what kind of asshole kills birds to demonstrate his domination of nature when he isn't hungry? On a spiritual level where one is lifting spirits to flight, what are we to think of a man who cuts off wings? Is this a statement that makes the dangerous attractive—or praises weakness?

One of the problems with the concept of art concerns external direction and response to feedback. When one is embedded in the web of circumstance, it is often difficult to remember that going with the flow is following one's truest nature. Your life is your art. It is more fun to be part of something legendary. Following your heart seems to lead to the greatest emotional rewards and even occasionally ties into fiscal returns if the investment in quality is great enough. Leaping outside the realms of conventionality continually results in growth if your basics are good enough to sustain you when confronting the unknown. The journey within eventually leads to exterior connections only faintly described by adventurers lacking in communicative ability. Research this well.

Chapter Eight

Seeing and Feeling the Aura

O NE'S AURA IS the subtle field of energy surrounding and generated by the human being, of which the thickest and heaviest part is called the body. I've researched quite a few different books on the aura and must point out that there is some of diversity in what people claim to be able to see. The aura as seen by a skilled healer who is guided by a spirit differs from that which is usually seen by the martial artist. The part which is easiest to see is light and denser than the air in which the body is immersed. It extends out from the body's surface approximately one-quarter to one-half inch on most people and is referred to as the functional or etheric body in the literature of Western mystics. On a powerful individual it may radiate up to ten times the norm.

The next layer out which can be easily seen if you stay relaxed is somewhat egg-shaped, colored by the fluxions of the hormone system, extends out a yard or so on intense people, and is called the emotional body or *nin* (spirit) in Japanese. It is said to have great healing and protective powers if dominated by the next two layers. It is a presence easily read and felt with practice. The fields at the edge of perception are called the *mental body* (socialized thought or learned self), the *energy field* (soul, avatar, or bridge power), and the *circumference of the personality* (realm of the archetypes, immortals, and inner deities as well as the connection to the universal or Void). I will discuss the subjective reality for an adventurer in these three realms of energy or power in the third book of this series.

Seeing into these fields of energy simply requires using your night vision in the daytime and two other easy abilities: 1. being in a relaxed, open state of mind, and 2. having enough control over your eyes to shift your focus in and out of 20/20 so that you can notice some phenomena you normally ignore. For example, where there is injury to the fields they will move more slowly and that creates a shadow or an opening in the field. There are critical points on the body that could almost be said to glow from the amount of energy that runs through them. Depending on the point's function it will pull or push energy into the fields around the body. In the martial arts some of these points are called pressure points, because if you whack them with a strong pressure you disrupt organs.

The relaxed individual glows in a different way from the uptight individual. Powerful and dangerous animals give off very different vibes than the dangerous and weak, or the powerful and playful. Certain character traits which can be seen in the aura with a lot of casual practice tend to predict first moves under stress that are simple enough to be survival mechanisms. It is useful to know when one is likely to take a stand, or is in love. I used to glow pink at ninja seminars because I was having so much fun and loved doing it. I'd taught Dr. Jon Kayne, the vice president of Bellvue College in Kansas, how to see auras and took him to a ninja seminar so he could put it to use, as it is easiest to see around intense performers. When he told me I was glowing pink, I almost fell down laughing. Pink is for pregnant girls in love, according to my experience.

Color predicts in funny ways as I just described, but the descriptions tend toward biology. When your hands become sensitive enough to feel and follow the points, there are opportunities for healing as well as serious harm. It takes experimentation on hundreds of bodies to get super-accurate, but if you can hit through a pine board you can miss by a little, and if you can break a patio block, you can miss by a lot.

When I was a college professor, I had psychometric data on all the managers who went through our Self-Analysis for Leadership course. I took a sample of one hundred volunteer managers and showed them how to "see" auras. Most were able to distinguish colors in the heat envelope or electrical fields surrounding the body within twenty minutes. The fourteen conventional perfectionists who weren't ever able to distinguish the differences or see anything going on at all were fun to observe as they, of course, thought everyone else was bonkers or hypnotized. This little evening exercise usually created some very interesting discussion. I usually finished this session with the following statement and question, "This has been around you all your life, but because it's subtle, it's very easy to miss or forget. What else have you been missing because you didn't know what to ask or chose not to learn?"

I consider statistics as proof of relationships, as do most scientists. Colors positively correlate with the Go Dai or chakra system and related scores on appropriate psychological inventories. It's not all significant but it's strong enough to be interesting. People normally don't have very bright auras. (This is also true in England, France, Germany, Spain, Brazil, South Africa and Japan.) Brightness seems to relate to energy. The colors shift a lot. People who meditate and people who do tai chi, chi kung, or taijutsu usually have bigger, brighter auras with easier-to-discern colors. Many entertainers have large bright auras. A blues singer puts out like a torch. It seems to relate to what we call charisma, but the media can't seem to define.

People who can't control their blink rate, who are color blind, who are significantly ($<.05$) more conventional, perfectionist, and rigid in their psychological make-up, or who try real hard won't see auras. That piece of information from a three-year study I couldn't get anyone to publish. Auras and retinal retention are completely different phenomena. See if you can get your retinal retention to change and move with the thoughts of the person you are observing. People who can go into relaxation response with their eyes open, who are (<.05) significantly more flexible, less conventional, and perfectionist, usually will see auric phenomena once shown how. It's really just a matter of using your binocular vision to shift your focus to one of greater dilation to take in more light. American Indian traditional healers refer to it as using "soft eyes."

Here's the method I usually use to show someone how to see auras for the first time:

1. Sit facing a friend or subject placed against a white, grey, or light violet background in a room with dimmable lights. You may have to experiment with the lighting. I prefer the lights to be dim, but not dark.

2. Have the subject hold a finger approximately six inches in front of their face. Go into relaxation response and focus on the finger, so that it is sharp and clear and their face is slightly out of focus or blurred.

3. Once your eyes get used to being slightly out of focus, look above their forehead and between their ears and shoulders. You'll probably get a thin corona of misty lighter color or white. Let your eyes shift out to about three inches above the head and then down around the shoulders. You'll probably get color. If you don't, have the subject close their eyes, breathe deeply, and think about something they really enjoy and like. Observe the shifts, particularly around the head. Ask the subject to pause, take a deep breath, and begin thinking about something they really dislike. Observe.

4. Memorize how you feel as you are doing this, not what you are doing. Play with it. Practice under different conditions. Practice makes it easier. Being in a relaxed or meditative state is also helpful.

This phenomenon is complex and varied. Body temperature, electro-chemical-biological fields, traits and intention, nutrition, and being able to see into the ultraviolet spectrum are all involved. Mystics and healers use the aura as a diagnostic device. Real martial artists have it as an ace up their sleeve regardless of their physical skills. Being able to see the aura and how energy moves through a person can be an enormous aid to the selection of fighting or teaching strategies as the descriptions given in Mikkyo and

Shingon Buddhism seem to be based on extensive empiricism.

This also can provide endless hours of entertainment and fun insights once you've mastered the eye trick so you can do it while you're moving. Don't take it too seriously or draw conclusions until you've "seen" many people under different circumstances. Some of the stuff I've seen written by supposed esoteric experts was way off the mark from my experience. *Caveat emptor* (let the buyer beware). I could usually verify what I was seeing by bringing in a student or friend. Not always trusting my own interpretation of esoteric matters, I highly recommend that you experiment and draw your own conclusions. Following are some things to look for with no guarantees of consistent replication.

I've noticed that when people do not believe what they are saying (an unkind person might regard this as lying), their body aura around the heart and along the shoulders will often flash a drab green. The ninjas refer to this as Negative Wind and associate it with misplaced idealism, which I've also seen described as jealousy. Auras often get redder and bigger with alcohol consumption. People with bright yellow auras tend to be assertive, not saintly. Indecisiveness and/or lack of integration may be shown by the body aura being very different from that around the head.

Bars, dances, airport terminals, churches, and other places where people congregate can be very educational when you can read intent and see auras. Most people can't hide their intent so being able to "see" it provides a beneficial non-verbal clue to the wise observer; for example, the darker shades and mixes of the primary colors—brown (inflated ego, needs to win), beige (dependence and cowardice), olive drab (lying and jealousy)—seem to indicate negative traits or character disorders. Healers also see the darker areas as blockages in energy flow. I've never seen a black aura as such except when watching an example of possession by a goddess. I've never seen a chakra either but they are very easy to feel. When you occult your fields to hide or project *chitta* (living energy that obeys your intent), you can make it pretty dark. The deep visionary thinkers put out some indigo that can look like black under the right conditions. I tend to put the black auras and plane crash or elevator fall tales into the teller-probably-flashes-olive-drab category or someone watching a death angel at work. Usually people who meditate will have a wider corona surrounding their bodies. If the energy moves in the brain, a result of meditation and certain types of prayer, the alpha wave cap may project out in an actual vertical halo effect (I have only seen this effect in church choir singers). Healers will often have little whirling balls in their auras like little stars and nebulas. I travel in some odd circles and visit some exotic places and keep my eye out. You should, too!

The first time I met ninja shidoshi Stephen Hayes was at his invitation to attend one of his Dayton dojo seminars (1982 or 1983). He was teaching what esotericists familiar with Japanese concepts refer to as the *Go Dai* (five great understandings) but in a way I'd never seen before. No mystical trappings, just directed meditations, specific body movements, and self-defense techniques that were incredibly powerful yet flowed. By the second day of this unique and earthy training, I noted that the coronas and auric fields surrounding the heads and shoulders of all fifty participants were now pinkish red or bright red rather than the usual wimpy mix you see in any typical gathering. I was impressed and intrigued. The ninjas could do something I couldn't do and furthermore could whip butt! My money was well spent.

The next seminar I was able to attend had the Wind as a topic, and many of the same people were present as well as new faces. By the second day all the participants had nice little apple-green auras and I distinctly remembered two-thirds of them were red the last time I'd seen them. These guys were jumping two chakras in months. Very interesting. A few in attendance noticed this phenomenon of light around the body when we were doing some exercises in handicapped light conditions. Hayes treated it very lightly and went on to other things. The next seminar addressed the Void, and I decided to take my friend and colleague Dr. Jon Kayne along, as he would make a good witness to some of my observations, being a clinical-type psychologist and statistician. By the third day the aura colors all matched the course content.

Kayne was able to see this also. *Folies á deux* (French expression for contagious craziness) confirmed.

I wrote a paper on the Go Dai, psychometrics, and archetypes that was greeted with such excitement by the journals that no one would publish it. Each one said the subject matter could be handled better by some other journal, which said, " It's not quite what we do. Send it to_____." I would occasionally show this paper to a friend. After collecting some more data and running the appropriate statistical tests I used it to obtain a Sc.D. from Eurotechnical Research University. I'm probably the world authority on the subject now.

One of the things that impressed me about Stephen Hayes in those early years was that as he moved through each stage of a technique, his aura flashed to the appropriate color corresponding to the body movement. He had definitely trained his intent. Sometimes he would shoot little rainbows out of the limbic regions of his head as he explained something. He'd trained as an actor and writer in college but fell in love with the machismo of the martial arts as he perceived them until he ran into Hatsumi. Acting, as well as dance, are two of the traditional Western paths to enlightenment as well as a ninja specialty necessary for information gathering in hostile or ambiguous situations. A spy may have to maintain a role for years, and his or her death can be the reward of a bad performance. Hayes already understood how to get into a part so the direction and shaping of intention was easy for him to understand, internalize, and teach in a dramatic and easily grasped manner. He's a brilliant teacher. He's got a great sense of humor when he's not being frustrated by Hatsumi or his own sense of righteousness. If you want to learn taijutsu of the spirit, Hayes is one of the round-eyes that can teach you. Particularly if you enjoy a more systematic, heroic, and formal approach to learning this ancient and chaotic tradition.

Many of the other high-level shidoshi teach more from the perspective of the *kihon hoppo* or basic moves. I prefer the Go Dai but then my perspective is more inclined to the esoteric and psychological. I am not interested in holding myself up as an exem-

117

plar of masterful taijutsu. There are many teachers of taijutsu who are much more demanding and thus better at the technical aspects than I. There is also a strong tendency to favor what you learn first as the basis for what follows. The ability to see and use information from your opponent's aura far transcends the simple kick, punch, or throw, no matter how beautifully and powerfully executed. Not all the shidoshi in Bujinkan are inclined toward the bioelectric or androgyny. After they age and lighten up a bit, they may enlarge their studies. In the Hoshinroshiryu, seeing and reading the aura is the kihon hoppo.

The first time I saw Hatsumi, he was running continuous bright, lime, neon green a foot wide and was so easy to see he would flash in bright sunlight. Now his aura runs white most of the time, at least when I've had the privilege to attend some function where he is teaching or when we could party together. I've seen him run every other color when doing taijutsu. Kevin Millis, who sees Hatsumi much more often than I do, has confirmed this observation of the White Dragon on his mountain.

One of Kevin's students is a Zen priest into shiatsu and massage. It's a privilege to get on his table. Since Bill has been working on Kevin, he shines like a Christmas tree. Sometimes the auric corona around the body looks a bit like the old movie scenes when the actors were shot against an outdoor movie backdrop. When I showed Ishizuka-sensei how to see auras, after his wife had demonstrated the tea ceremony for me, he asked me if Hatsumi knew how to do this. I said I didn't know if he knew how to see them, but he certainly had one that was easy to see and he'd be a good subject to study, which made Ishizuka (The Steel Man) laugh with delight.

Feeling the body's electrochemical fields is relatively easy. First raise your hands in front of you with your palms together. Relax, breathe slowly. Separate your hands and wave the fingers of your right hand slowly past the palm of your left. You may feel a faint sensation as if the palm were brushed by a feather. Pay attention to the palm, not the hand that is waving. You may have to close your eyes. Move the waving hand away until you no longer feel the sensation. Move it back in. Switch hands. Notice the difference in sensitivity and handedness. The Chinese refer to this polarity as yin and yang. There are pictures of Rumiko doing this exercise in Stephen Hayes' Ohara books on ninjutsu.

Find someone else to play this with. Run your palms over their body at an inch or so distance. Move away. See what you feel. Come closer. See what you get. Start paying attention to what other people feel like in various situations. Pay attention to what you feel when you are around them. Practice distancing. Learn what you can from it. Don't rationalize the feelings, just build your catalog. Ninjas have interesting exercises like dodging fists and swords and shuriken blindfolded. (You start slow with padded weapons and work up to speed.) In the Hoshinroshiryu we observe our leaders and lovers. Healers identify blocked meridians, damaged chakras, and other potentials for disease. Each requires a great deal of sensitivity to rather subtle sensations. Remember blind Master Po of the glowing cataracts in the sixties television serial "Kung Fu."

Seeing the aura requires relaxed concentration. I have run into a few people who do it with considerable effort and the occasional "psychic" of genetic luck. I think it's easier if you learn how to relax into it. The just-try-harder types don't seem to have much of a success rate. When you can "see" other people's auras or spirits and have practiced "feeling" until you can trust your catalog, you will find that your sense of humor as well as compassion will have to expand if you want to maintain all of your acquaintances. This exercise provides a gateway to greater intuition skills such as empathy and telepathy and is considered a great boon by the healers who have mastered the process. If your lifestyle requires quickly identifying people who seem to be too good to be true, I throw in this little bone—a consistently grey aura is often indicative of a bullshitter in the thinner spread of the material world. Check it out.

Chapter Nine

Healing

MEDICAL PRACTITIONERS ARE not so secretive about chi kung, as they tend not to be interested in the darker side of its application. As power is derived from the shadow intuition or id, they usually aren't very good with it. Most of their training is with the intellect and memory, so they must resort to the knife for surgery or the acupuncture needle for generation. Practitioners of preventative medicine like chiropractors tend to have more skill, particularly after a few years of practice. It's all written down, has been for centuries. Many of the great karate masters have stated that to attain real greatness as a practitioner of karate you must become a healer. Most people don't have the clit or balls to go for it. Besides, it's dangerous.

If you don't know your meridians you're going to have one hell of a time figuring out how to effectively use chi. At the shidoshi training that Hatsumi held in Ishizuka's dojo during the celebration of his thirtieth year as grandmaster of the Togakure Ryu, he informed everyone there that if they really wanted to become accomplished at ninjutsu they must learn to think and study like medical doctors. There are many good books around now on acupuncture, shiatsu, and if you must, dim mak (*Butoku-den, Dim Mak*, Bernola and Morris, 1993). Knowledge of anatomy is essential to understanding yourself as well as dissecting others. In the long run you'll get a lot more use out of alternative medical skills than fighting skills. Applying chi kung to healing is one of the so-called *siddhi* or magics associated with enlightenment. Reiki, medical chi kung, shiatsu, homeopathy, and therapeutic touch are all based on the principles of harmonizing the flow of life energy to speed or restore healing energy as opposed to curing. Once you have learned how to generate and move energy through your own body it is a simple procedure to offer this blessing to others. You don't have to be deeply religious in the mundane sense. Practically anyone can give someone else a little blast of energy. I've been told by Crystal Kroll-Young that in Canada where therapeutic touch is part of the training for most nurses, no hospital staffed with TT nurses has ever been sued for malpractice. The trick is in intention.

Shiatsu, one of the Japanese massage therapies, is based on manipulation of the body's energy points and meridians, as is acupuncture. If you have chi there is no need for needles and microwattage since you provide the energy. All of the strikes in ninjutsu when applied properly are directed toward meridians, kinesiology release points, or acupuncture points *(tsubo)*. I've been told they are different, but if they are it's in degree more than placement. (Dr. Michael Fenster and I are researching fifty of the ryu's recommended points of retaliation *[kyusho]* from both the Eastern and Western medical perspective. We published a manual showing thirty-eight of these points after identifying them in four other systems.) If you've learned how to absorb and move energy a ninpo workout is like getting rather violent massage combined with chiropractic manipulation—one of the reasons why Hatsumi says the practice of taijutsu alone can bring enlightenment. Chi kung is a body skill.

If your partner is inept, you may get to work on your self-healing skills. If your partner is very inept or you haven't learned to go with the flow—a trivialized statement that has many levels of meaning—you can take or give yourself serious damage and get to meet an expensive and disapproving physician. Relaxation and good intentions are essential to high-level ninjutsu; that is one of the reasons the angry individuals tend to leave the art. They can't loosen up enough to do taijutsu without getting hurt. I have heard seminar attendees complain that their girlfriends are better at shiatsu massage than some of the ninja teachers. It takes a powerful soft hand.

In my discussion of kundalini in chapter three, I describe some of the dangers of being stiff-necked. I received an energy blast to the major meridians while standing nearly motionless, doing something that is supposed to be pleasing and relaxing. I fell to my knees and threw up, and it took six years and some help to heal. Take an energy blow when you're off balance, unaligned, frustrated, and angry from the full-body movement of whatever training partner has slammed you. . . . Your bones will knit eventually. Do some of the full extension blows and kicks when you're stiff and uptight and see what happens to your body. I saw Mark Kenworthy attempt a power mule kick out of a roll without warming up. He rolled around screaming as the muscles and ligaments tore loose in his quadriceps. He kicks very hard automatically because he trained for many years in karate. The bruises from internal damage went from his knee to his groin. His wasn't a steroid accident. Run hot angry emotions through your meridians and see if you like the migraine feeling. All fear and anger is an attempt by the social self to prevent change. Let the cosmos decide. Study on this.

When I was about twenty-five, I was living in Los Angeles on Manhattan Beach and decided to join the Los Angeles Police Department. They were helpful, as not too many college graduates/veterans are interested in police work. The physical at that time consisted of three X-rays: the head, chest, and legs. They took seven of me. When I asked the doctor why, he informed me that practically every bone in my body had suffered at least a hairline fracture: football, boxing, wrestling, jujitsu, karate, judo, kung fu, bar brawls, falls, car wrecks—an exciting life of near misses but considerable contact. They weren't going to take me, as I'd be pensioned out with arthritis by the time I was thirty-five.

When I was around thirty-eight and living a sedentary academic life, I dropped my daughter as I was picking her up because of the arthritic pain in my thumbs. She probably weighed less than sixty pounds. I'm forty-eight now, have no arthritis, no pains, and feel great. I place the blame for this rapid decline on returning to the martial arts, meditatively studying chi kung and ninjutsu, and practicing hoshin while having people half my age beat on my body twice a week. When the flesh is weak but the spirit is willing, regeneration can indeed take place. That's the way of endurance.

You can speed the process of healing or regeneration by stimulating the cell structure of the injured area with chi. In alchemy this is called transmutation or transubstantiation. In Methodism we call it the laying on of hands and in ninjutsu, as well as Tibetan Buddhism, it is one of the ways of taming demons. A thoroughly bad person requires a heavy healing hand. Those of us with a more intellectual inclination toward the "way of death" or transformation of the self (which includes the study of disease) are easily sidetracked by the healthful benefits of self-protection. I'm happy to watch the youngsters whip on each other; I know what damage feels like. At my age, I'd much rather coach than experience.

Therapeutic touch is augmented by a knowledge of anatomy. It is particularly helpful if you study shiatsu and the acupuncture meridians so you can move energy most easily through another's body. Nurses are very good at it, if they are familiar with loving feelings, anatomy, and positive thought. Only a few male physicians seem to be aware of its existence. You might read Bernie Siegel or Larry LeShan. The magazine from Pacific Rim Publications called WuShu *Qi Qong* may stimulate thought.

When we were studying the effects of shiatsu at Hillsdale College as part of our hoshin regimen, we discovered ways to reduce pain, speed healing, and increase or reduce strength. There are techniques for controlling menstrual cramps and PMS and for energizing the body. In the West shiatsu can be compared to kinesiology. I remember the beautiful young actress-in-training, Suzanne Carlson, giving us a lesson in intention: One afternoon we were discussing what point manipulations seemed to work and what seemed to have little or no effect in reducing menstrual cramps. One technique we'd found in an old Korean medical text on massage had general acceptance with the women in the class. Suzanne was saying it didn't work on her roommate at all. In fact, she had worse pains when Suzanne worked on her. I asked Suzanne how she felt about her roomie, and she expressed extreme dislike. After laughing heartily, I suggested that when she worked on her roommate to confine her thoughts to healing or maintain neutrality. When she did that, the techniques were effective.

The lesson in this is you get what you project. The healing energy of the open heart is light green in color. Any of the lighter colors will work; pink, white, bright yellow, and green are considered the best, but it's an individual thing relating to the chakras or Go Dai. Usually where there is an energy block or injury the molecular friction will heat up and/or thicken the area's energy field. It's like a stickiness in the air. Often just brushing your hand through it will begin its dissipation, and as the flow returns to normal the increased energy in the area will lead to a return of normal function. Skill levels can be developed from direct manipulation to healing from a distance, using the body's electrical fields in preference to the manipulation of muscle and bone. I have "watched" healers of great skill use these techniques and been on the receiving end to test their efficacy at Association for Humanistic Psychology conventions. It's another skill helpful in avoiding the scalpel as well as the sword. A study published in the International Society for the Study of Subtle Energies and Energy Medicine journal *Subtle Energies* (Vol. 1, No. 1, 1990), in which the placebo effect was eliminated by using a double-blind study experimental format, showed an increase of healing speed by a factor of ten in the subjects exposed to non-contact therapeutic touch or external chi kung. Learning energy skills strikes me as an essential component of martial practice, from being a booster to first aid to an adjunct to strategy.

Self-protection might include the idea that the organs of your body are part of your self. The wellness and prevention movements are not the blathering of airheads. A simple shiatsu technique controls and can eliminate tachycardia. Look up what your pharmacist or surgeon consider a cure.

When I was a medic in the army and practicing *O'Neill Quick Kill* (military application of combatic jujitsu emphasizing hand strikes and snap kicks, developed for the British Special troops by the Gurkhas and a former member of the Hong Kong police in World War Two), a friend who was a sergeant in the infantry and practiced a form of karate used to beat his knuckles on the cast-iron fences that surrounded our *kasernes* (barracks in Germany). He wanted me to break the knuckles in his hands so that the bone callous would be even thicker. I did it for him, since I knew he'd never play the violin and it made him happy. Miyamoto Musashi says that he dislikes hard hands. Art requires sensitivity. Energy moves through soft hands. Women tend to be better at healing.

Here's an exercise for you to try out.

Think about a time when you were relaxed and happy. Think about a time when you really loved someone or something. Put the care and affection you feel into your hands. Handle something alive, even a plant. I've potted plants that are ten years old and still doing fine under my sporadic care. I mow the lawn in my bare feet. Linda thinks I'm crazy. Her plants die with great regularity. According to the most recent medical research on chi kung published by the Institute for Noetic Science, these ancient and once-secret breath and movement techniques revitalize the endocrine/chakra systems, which correspond to the Go Dai. Practitioners live long lives without senility. The practices reduce or prevent hardening of the arteries as well as stimulate the central nervous system. I recently had the honor of meeting with Eurotechnical Research University's School of Polemikology, Rockwell College's Chinese Martial Arts department heads. Except for Brendan Lai, they are all in their seventies and it would be extremely difficult to place any of them older than fifty. Dr. Yuang (seventy-five, All China Wu Shu Champion and chi kung practitioner) still has black hair. None of their wives looked older than forty. Chi kung has shown a phenomenal effect and unique function in preventing and treating disease; maintaining good health; increasing and promoting intelligence; resisting aging and retaining youthful appearance and body movement; raising working energy and efficiency; and strengthening and arousing the interior latent energy of the body. The therapeutic effect of qiqong is particularly noteworthy in the treatment of diseases afflicting the digestive, respiratory, cardiovascular, and nervous systems.

I strongly suspect the exaggerated descriptions of the healing powers of the ancients worked as a rhetorical device, but I can easily see the wisdom of applying energy methods where appropriate. I trust my own experience and recommend you try it out yourself. It's a lot slower than surgery and seldom requires anesthetic. Don't rely on martial applications; try some different flavors of bodywork. The basic material is the same but the application is quite different.

Following is a meditation used to increase one's ability to use therapeutic touch and expand consciousness. You are expected to have mastered deep belly breathing, the Secret Smile, and quieting your mind as described in chapter five on meditation. This is to be done in the sage position, seiza, or upright in a chair. Once you are in a deep state of relaxed balance and your breathing has settled, have a friend read this to you as a directed meditation.

Picture yourself walking along a beach. *(Pause)* As you walk you are beginning to shrink. This does not frighten you, as it is very interesting. You quickly find yourself going down to the size of the sand grains upon which a moment before you were treading. *(Pause)* Soon the grains appear as mountains and then separate into worlds unto themselves as you continue to shrink down to the molecular level. *(Pause)* As you continue to shrink and slip between the atoms, each atom seems a star or diamond in the emptiness and you can faintly see the energy lines that connect them like a web or net flung out of points of light. *(Pause)*

You continue to shrink and fall through space, flying like a bird though you are in a vacuum, eventually approaching a point of light you pick from the web. As you grow closer it begins to appear as a world, and then our beloved Earth as seen from space.

(Pause) You continue to approach, huge in comparison but still shrinking rapidly as you enter the atmosphere and fly down through the blue sky over ocean waves toward a sandy beach. You float up to a likely landing spot and hit the position you like to use for meditation. You open your eyes.

Practice this until it becomes easy to shrink your consciousness and send it out scouting along the energy lines or the spaces between. I think the therapeutic touch applications will become evident when you are able to project your intent into your hands and beyond. Some people pick this up with remarkable speed, and for others it doesn't seem to have much effect beyond being an interesting visualization. This exercise can be considered a preparation and aid to achieving astral projection as well as a tool for achieving more precise and subtle healing. Play with this, as it is an exercise congruent with more than one esoteric tradition.

When you have trained your mind to project an intention, such as liking or alertness, you can move that projection through the practice of chi kung concentration into another person's aura or into the proper meridian. Working on your therapeutic touch prolongs your life as a protector and healer, as well as increases your power as a teacher.

Chapter Ten

Teaching Esoteric Strategy at the College Level

or

Founding an American Ryu
to compete with Ninjutsu

I N 1981 I took an administrative position at Hillsdale College in southern Michigan. It was a new experience for me as the college was small, private, and conservative. I was used to teaching at large, public, and liberal colleges. My job was an instructor in social psychology for the Dow Leadership Development Center, which meant working with managers from all over the world every other week to do psychological assessments and teach teamwork, problem-solving, and people skills in a workshop setting. After a year had passed and the responsibilities became routine, I also took over the Speech Department, as the administration of the college had decided to eliminate the program. This struck me as fatuous for a liberal arts college so I volunteered to teach all the courses required for a communication minor on a rotating basis. It wasn't part of my job description but I'd taught speech at Penn State, Wayne State, and the University of Windsor. Since the administration wasn't willing to pay me for the class but was willing to charge the students, I taught the courses as if they were graduate seminars. I liked the students and it was fun.

The work was sedentary, and my second wife, Linda, was an excellent cook and lover so I began to put on weight. After reaching 260 pounds on a light-boned, six-foot frame I decided to start working out again (twelve years later I'm at 180). I'd quit the study of martial arts for eight years before I signed up for the college's tae kwan do course. The instructor, Brian Anderson, was very competent, but I quickly realized that tae kwan do was more sport than combat and for someone of my age and condition too hard on the joints, particularly the hips. I've also never been particularly fond of *kata* (forms) except for tai chi, and one-point sparring bores me to tears. One of the red belts noticed that when I couldn't perform a particular tae kwan do maneuver I'd slip in something that worked for me. He asked me what I was doing and I replied "Jujitsu." His response changed my life. "Teach me," he said with a grin.

Campbell "Camper" Walker was extremely skilled in the kicking techniques and also *nunchakus* (Okinawan karate weapon developed in China). As I taught him throwing and joint locking, he taught me different footwork and "karate sticks." We spent a lot of time figuring out how to defeat each other's favorite techniques. As we were more friends than student and teacher, a lot of our interaction included talking about books, life in general, and what was important to him at his age. He was a guest at my home and reciprocated. I was having such a good time playing warrior with Camper that I decided to systematize what I had learned over the years into an intelligent, challenging course. At the end of the year I'd broken down the belt system into a self-defense course plus readings which would take approximately six semesters to achieve a black belt if you were smart and normally athletic. When I showed it to Camper he informed me I'd left out the most important part.

"Your mind," he said. "It's not the techniques but how you teach them, the meditation, the strategy, sharing your thoughts and feelings. That's what's important! You always tell me the truth. You never bullshit. Most of the professors here are so full of themselves and their subjects, you can't really learn from them. You treat us like we matter. You've got to get that loving what you are and doing into the course."

I was stunned. He went on. "Everybody wants to meet a real master and study with them. When I tell my friends what I've been doing the last year they're so envious. You've got to put the hidden meanings and all the psychological stuff in the course. We'll use that; most of us will never have to be in a physical fight once we get out of school. We have to learn strategy! It's so much fun!"

After being chased around by a smart, dangerous, twenty-two-year-old for a year, his request had more than ordinary appeal. The trick would be how to get the right stuff into a package acceptable to modern Americans while still making them able to defend themselves physically as well as mentally in ways appropriate to their environment. I may have seemed masterful to Camper, but why not expose young students to the ancient masters, real masters, and professionals, not just a hobbyist like myself. The syllabus in my head got a lot more interesting. Things that I'd seen over the years and wanted to experience myself combined with a basic core of exercises and techniques associated with transformation of consciousness. Modern hoshinjutsu was born out of that discussion.

Replication is the heart of science. Camper had a young Alaskan friend who wanted to study with me. His name was Steve Noonkesser. He was a history major and very analytical, good with computers, and loved playing Dungeons and Dragons. His joining our little circle made the next semester very interesting. Teaching should also be learning, and Steve, having grown up in Alaska with Eskimos, had some very interesting perspectives concerning man's place in nature. We began to integrate some of the techniques he'd learned from his Indian friends into the course. I began to study and practice chi kung and Iyengar yoga, which amplified the Zen practice I'd been doing on and off for years. I learned how to dungeon-master and we added role playing to our strategy sessions as mental exercises.

Camper and I had boiled down hundreds of techniques to what we thought were the most effective requiring the least amount of strength. Steve, because he was physically powerful, became our guinea pig. He also encouraged the introduction of weapons at a much lower belt level than Camper and I had discussed. We decided that improvised weapons and easily concealed weaponry made more sense for modern times so we lifted *hanbo* (cane) and chain *(kusari fundo)* techniques from ninjutsu for our basics. We derived our warm-up exercises from yoga, chi kung, and tai chi. We decided to wear black gi's instead of white to differentiate ourselves from tae kwan do and emphasize our non-sport, self-protection orientation.

We went through one more step. I wanted a student who was smart, small, athletic, and exemplified the conservative, status-seeking, upwardly mobile, middle-class young people typical of Hillsdale College. Someone who had never been in a real fight in his life. Enter Randy Reising, ex-high-school football player and gymnast, and gentleman about town. Randy became the final authority as to what techniques were kept or dropped. As he had no experience and was learning everything through new eyes, he became our best critic and most proficient practitioner. We combed through the martial arts literature, paying particular attention to the techniques recommended for women and the elderly. We'd take something like a hip throw and see how many variations of it we could find in different martial arts. Then we would take it all apart and develop variations on the basic theme based on utility, kinesiology, or escalation of pain, damage, and energy flow, saving the nastiest techniques for the higher levels as opposed to the more athletic. We called these "fifth-picture moves" because in many of Hatsumi's Japanese books on ninpo he'd show four pictures breaking down a technique and the fifth was usually something only a truly creative and nasty person would do to another human being in the midst of a fight.

I submitted the syllabus to the physical education department. The course was accepted, and the next semester we had twenty willing scholars. Little did we know what we had started. Each student was given a packet of readings, copies of the written exam to be completed after reading *The Book of Five Rings* by Miyamoto

Musashi, and a list of techniques they were expected to master for an A in the course. Camper graduated and Steve and Randy became my assistant instructors. The class met for two hours every Friday afternoon as a way to guarantee only interested people would sign up. We were given the use of the dance studio but often took the class outside so people could practice their techniques on varying surfaces.

During our search of the literature we discovered Stephen Hayes. Hayes is one of the first Westerners to be trained in the traditional ninja life-ways as taught by Grandmaster Masaaki Hatsumi of the Togakure Ryu of Japan. When I discovered he lived a day away in Ohio, I called him and he graciously invited me to attend a special weekend workshop for his black belts and others. I was deeply impressed by the skills taught and even more by how they were taught. Hayes used directed meditations, music when appropriate, emphasized stretching and body movement, and, most interesting for me, connected attitude/intent to technique. It was apparent that the ninjas with their 800-year-old warrior tradition had already accomplished for the professional what we were trying to put together for the hobbyist. That weekend eventually led to the inclusion of many ninja ideas in our course, as the ninja reputation as the "ultimate warriors" is based in the reality of their training. As we began to experience some of the side effects of enlightenment it was comforting to know there were people out there who were even crazier than we were. Taijutsu as taught by the Bujinkan is definitely a path to mushin. One must train the intent before one can release it.

One of the things about the martial arts that always annoyed me in my own studies was the imposed hierarchy of master over student or teacher/leader as omnipotent source of correct knowledge. As an intelligent observer of many things I found that rule hard to ingest. Realizing that the *sensei* (one who has gone before) served as a model, I wanted our dojo climate to be more relaxed, open, and fun than is usual to more traditional systems. Play is important to learning. The closest to my particular ideal have been the various Togakure Ryu Bujinkan Ninpo dojos in which

I'd trained. Every semester I would give a lecture on how one should act when visiting other training halls—depth of bows, courtesy, belts and sashes, flags, shrines, and all that. I'd been in more than a few over the years. Then I'd point to the light switch on the far wall and say, "If you feel you have to worship someone or something in here, I'd suggest the source of electricity because that's as close to magic as we'll get. To me this is all science."

As most people get started in the martial arts because they fear others, I felt it necessary to do everything possible to reduce fear and instill curiosity. All anger is rooted in fear of loss. I wanted to encourage flexibility of mind, body, and spirit and felt that could best be accomplished in a democratic atmosphere. I wanted my students to be relaxed and calm so we always opened with a meditation and some stretching. I wanted the women to advance in the system, so upper body strength techniques were minimized. Taijutsu, jujitsu techniques for older people, and chi kung held the key to accomplishing that particular riddle. It was felt at that time that the women would have a gentling effect. Both sexes have the opportunity to know each other much better, reducing shyness and fear, and increasing confidence. Sexual tension keeps everyone alert, as there is something arousing in making the beautiful dangerous. The other differences were much greater emphasis on training the mind and particularly the emotions, early use of pick-up weapons, and application of strategy. Women make very sneaky opponents. (The Japanese strategists regard them as personifying treachery. The Chinese would wound/bind their feet from birth so concubines could not develop complete use of chi, nor flee their fate.)

Five kyu belt levels were developed using the Go Dai as a basis, as well as five black belt levels that also required study and achieving rank in other martial systems to test one's survival and intelligence gathering skills. Ninpo, having the least weaknesses, became the favored other system to explore unless we could find a legitimate kung fu master. Each belt had an associated series of readings, yogic exercises, healing practices, and specific techniques and principles to be mastered before going on to the next belt package. Students always had a good idea of where they were in the system. Higher-level ranks were assigned students to bring along and could not advance until their students had reached the appropriate level, guaranteeing they learned how to teach. Teaching is the only universal marker of a leader.

Trapping and woodsmanship as well as modern weapons familiarization at the local range became part of the curriculum. We included a heavier emphasis on chi kung and meditation as well as a greater emphasis on esoteric self-protection as greater skills began to emerge in what the ancients referred to as *siddhi* (the eight learned magics) and we called weird science; strategy from numerous sources both East and West; and greater emphasis on play, realizing that when the adrenals took over in a real fight, the spirit would emerge. We put in a fire-walking party at the end of each semester and held annual trophy raids on the fraternities and sororities during Greek Week, as one of the visiting ninjutsu instructors, John Porter, enjoyed that sort of thing. One of the girls in the system was so good at her stealth techniques that she would write me letters on the college president's personal stationery and had a collection of her target fraternity banners in consecutive years.

Eventually three hundred students achieved at least the first two belts as part of their physical education requirement. We had a pile of data from their experiences—aura reading, telempathy, telekinetics with energy, telepathy, far sensing, survival of falls and electrical accidents, chi development, shared dreams, healing of endless nicks and bruises, escapes from and capture of thugs, and accusations of witchcraft by the fundamental Christian Inter Varsity student group. Dr. Jon Kayne, a clinical psychologist, would test the black belts on Rhine cards and for precognition. They all scored higher than normal expectations. (It appears to me that the psychic researchers are looking for the light in the wrong places.) We never got levitation but Skippy Lepire developed some altitude and hang times that put him in a class with Air Jordan. In five years we tried out everything we could think of or that somebody else described well enough for us to take on. I paid for instructors in ninjutsu, karate, and kung fu to come and give guest lectures and demonstrations. We would troop off to take seminars by instructors in other arts who were invariably surprised to get a gaggle of outsiders attending their demos. Such are the dangers of offering public training. We did all the things a bunch of bright smart people are going to try if given the opportunity. We had a ball.

Of the three hundred, only four were malignant enough that I quit teaching them and finally drove them away. We treated all the siddhi (will discuss the siddhi more in the chapter "Magic, Crystals, Talismans and Swords") as benefits rather than goals and worked on our art and energy. Most of my students applied their new understandings to their professions as opposed to their new hobby of scientific mugging. Some were even horrified that they couldn't get out of the class without passing the physical measures at a standardized level of expectation of being able to quickly end a fight by winning.

After I left Hillsdale College to consult with the Engine Division of General Motors, a number of students enrolled specifically to get hoshin, not bad for a one-credit gym course. I'm teaching it again now that I've accomplished my primary goals in ninpo. I needed to make some high-level friends. I didn't seem to find any in business, academia, or church. I felt it was necessary to achieve a master's license in a different art from hoshin as it struck me as hubris and self-promotion to take that title on without proof from a legitimate lineage. I was able to do that by relying on what we had researched and developed at Hillsdale College. I consider hoshinjutsu to be a close but honed-down approximation of the ancient ryus as well as a modern introductory course that enables students to enter the world of the true or combatic martial artist without fear, and to have the confidence to follow their hearts far beyond the techniques represented by sport, the color of their obis, or the limitations of their instructors. Hoshin provides a vehicle for attaining the advantages of flow or enlightened movement without the risk of surviving endless battles with others.

It forces the issue to conquering one's own fears while entering unknown territory in the company of friends. Creation of this system for American martial artists was recognized by the World Martial Arts Hall of Fame and was the reason for my election to that august body. I am, and will be forever, grateful to my students for teaching me the way.

Chapter Eleven

Exchanges with Interesting People

THIS CHAPTER IS a little parody of Gurdjieff's conversations with great men, with vignettes or descriptions of people who've impressed or inspired me in the martial arts and related arenas.

First I'll describe two conversations with Masaaki Hatsumi and their after-effects. I was walking across the big quad at the Girl Scout camp near Kettering, Ohio, where Steve used to hold the Ninja Festival when I felt Hatsumi behind me. I turned around and he was coming out of the dinner hall with Nagato, Kan (I think), and Jack Hoban. I waited until they crossed the seventy yards or so to see what the grandmaster wanted of lowly white-belt me. This was 1987 and I'd been wearing glasses since the late seventies. The usual middle-age astigmatism. Hatsumi grabbed my hands, looked into my eyes, and asked me what I thought about ninjutsu. I told him I was enjoying the training enormously and felt that what he was demonstrating was of great value. He would ask me a question and Jack Hoban and Nagato would translate back and forth. He did not let go of my hands.

I noticed he was drawing energy from me and I started to laugh and draw energy from him. He was startled, grinned at me, and began to pull harder. I reciprocated and we began to run a circle of energy through each other's arms. Jack and the shihans did not notice what Hatsumi and I were doing. We were both giggling like schoolboys playing a prank and trying to maintain the conversation as if nothing esoteric were happening. We finished our exchange. He released my hands and walked off with his entourage. I turned toward my bunkhouse and noticed that I could see every leaf in the trees with clarity. My eyes were healed. I didn't need my glasses anymore. This lasted for over five years. They've weakened a little since 1987 but not enough for me to elect for glasses. (I take ginseng, and work on my breath, and palm when I remember.) When I saw him again at the Los Angeles Tai Kai (annual gathering of the Bujinkan) the next year, I thanked him for my better vision; he laughed and said, "I have very young energy."

Kevin Millis and I were in Noda City, Japan, for advance training. "The Boss" had invited us over to his house for some *sake* (rice wine) and conversation on a cold winter's night. Hatsumi had warmed up some sake on his little burner and we were bundled up among his collection of books and medical equipment. There was a jug of clear liquid with a snake dissolving in it on a shelf over my head, alongside the autographed poster of 1960s German sex symbol/movie star Elke Sommers. One of Hatsumi's dogs was trying to get to know me. The atmosphere was relaxed and comfortable. Hatsumi poured sake and when he handed me mine there was a tuft of dog hair pressed to the lip of the cup. (He'd reached over at some point and pulled a little off the beast, then neatly arranged it.) I thanked him for his gracious offer, turned the little cup and drank, swiped off the hair unobtrusively with a finger, and extended the cup for more. (He was testing my ability to deal with the unexpected, as well as checking my tolerance.)

We talked about various things, and then I decided to have some fun with him and see what he knew about *yidam*. Yidam are Tibetan warrior vampires, according to Chögyam Trungpa. Their particular task in life is the protection of the righteous. I asked Kevin to translate very carefully for me. He said he'd try.

I then said, "In the West, we have some very old customs concerning how to treat people who can work with energy. These traditions were designed specifically for those who could draw energy. We used to hunt them down, drive a wooden stake through their hearts, cut off their heads, and bury their remains at a crossroad. We call them vampires and they were much feared as you can imagine from the treatment. Yet I notice in Buddhism that people with many of the same characteristics of the legendary vampire are regarded as enlightened saints. Could you explain that to me?"

Kevin struggled with it. Hatsumi looked at me with a perplexed expression, suddenly stood up, walked over to a book stack on our right, and pulled out a beautiful collection of woodcuts. He said, "Here are some very nice thirteenth-century prints. Would you like to look at them?" The topic was closed. The prints weren't about vampires. It's not nice to joke about vampires around "the Boss." About a year later one of Nagato's students, a rather naive young sandan, informs me that Stephen Hayes is teaching vampire arts. Sorry, Steve, it's probably my fault. Hatsumi and I are the only real vampires I've noticed. There are a lot of politics in ninjutsu, but if you follow your heart everything that is said about the ultimate warriors can be found in the Togakure Ryu.

Sherm Harrell is a shichidan in Isshinryu Karate who has a dojo in Carson City, Iowa. Once a year he holds a seminar in Parma, Michigan, at Alandale Acres. His story, as told to me, is that his daughters were killed in a car crash. He withdrew from teaching and went into his cow barn and studied the scrolls given to him by his famous Okinawan teacher, Shimabuku. After two years of self-study he emerged with what he called *Jutedo* (soft hand way). It's a system of energy use attacking the meridians and balance points of the body and is a great improvement on how karate is typically taught. To the uninformed eye, it is a way of throwing people by striking them. It's very powerful and lots of fun to learn. I always make my students attend Sherm's seminars with me. He's a great teacher and usually wears his tattered white *obi* (belt). Andy Tucker, a shodan in hoshinjutsu as well as a black belt in tae kwan do, was sitting next to me putting on his tabi and said, "These karate guys are really old. Look at that old white belt in the crew cut having a cigarette. Do you think they really have something to show us?"

After Sherm finished his smoke, he came in, formally started the class, and began to demonstrate some of the most punishing techniques I'd ever seen on his assistant instructor, who spent the next hour or so flying through the air and landing on his butt or whatever got to the ground first. It was a great display of relaxed power. I was happy that we spent a lot of time on falling and rolling. Watching Andy handle his cognitive dissonance was fun. Sherm talked a lot about energy use and keeping soft through the techniques. The karate people were having trouble grasping the concepts, but my students jumped right on those bones of wisdom. They could see by his aura that he knew what he was doing when it came to moving chi around.

Sherm had gone through the kundalini on his own with no idea as to what was happening to him. He thought he was going crazy but knew in his heart that whatever was happening was for the best and he'd just have to ride it out. (Ex-Marines are tough.) He was still getting severe headaches after demos. He ran mostly yang energy, so we went outside and I showed him some of the chi kung techniques for bleeding off excess energy to the head. I sent him some articles from the Chinese National Chi Kung Institute on how to run the orbits. He sent me back a nice letter praising my students. Since he has only promoted two black belts in twenty years of teaching, that was high praise indeed.

Sherm spent many years on the *makiwara* (wrapped posts or wall hangers used for striking practice) and has the gnarly hands and feet to prove it. I watched him use soft sand palm techniques to break three patio blocks that were not separated. He then used soft techniques to break the middle block of five without breaking the two above or the two below. We then got to break a patio block using the same method. He showed a girl of eleven how to do it and she did it effortlessly. The hard breakers had a hell of a time. I did my patio block blindfolded. It was an eye-opener.

Sherm pointed out that once you learned the soft-hand techniques, all hard breaking was good for was reminding you about your arthritis on cold mornings. As a farmer in Iowa, he has a deep understanding of cold mornings. He's not a mystic, he's just real good at what he does.

Shihan Kevin Millis and I are good friends and often share our thinking and reactions to things and events around us. I think of myself as a fairly down-to-earth, middle-aged, middle-class college professor with Midwest values. I was visiting with Kevin and his parents near Malibu and asked him one afternoon what being around me was like. He said, "Being around you is like being around a Martian. You are a Midwest Mork with no Mindy in sight." I was saddened to hear that, as I thought I was learning to fit into the California Lifestyle. I was even beginning to like the Lakers and contemplating learning to rollerblade in Venice.

The Midwest Association of Humanistic Psychologists holds a convention in Indianapolis every year. I try to go if it's convenient and I have the money, or if the presenters look interesting. There are usually many healers and bodyworkers performing their art. I like to attend their seminars. It's a weakness of mine. Maybe I should have been a massage therapist.

In 1990 I went to two day-long certification granting seminars. The first was called "The Healing Process: Exploring Bodymind Integration." The teachers were two white witches into *Reiki* (Japanese energy work). One was Meg Blanchet-Cole, who obviously had a background in yoga, and the other was Barbara Allen, an R.N. with considerable chiropractic experience. We all sat down in a circle on our pillows. I had cleverly arranged to sit next to Meg, who is stunning and exudes a strong white aura. I noticed that she was blocking energy between her shoulder blades and reached over to hit the shiatsu points that would release it. She said, "Don't touch me!" I politely backed off.

The group was asked to introduce themselves and their specialties. It was heavily laced with bodyworkers of all sorts. I could learn a lot here. When it came my turn I introduced myself as "Dr. Morris, a fourth-degree black belt in Bujinkan Ninpo, and it is so nice to be a vampire here at play with all you nice people." The look of horror on Meg's face was well worth the price of admission. I paired off with a bodyworker named Sue from Chicago who was married to a martial artist, and we had a good time blowing out each other's circuits.

The next exercise involved feeling body energy around the chakras and we broke into triads. My group consisted of Meg's husband and an amazing girl who had walked across the Middle East as a teenager and eventually wound up learning energy work from Aborigines in Australia. She said, "I've never seen anyone like you before. All your energy is radiating from your head."

"That's what you're supposed to do with your sexual energy," I replied. "You move it up to your head so you can think with it. Then you can send it where it's needed."

"Oh, yeah. Send it to your feet." I did as she commanded. She was intrigued. "Send it to your chest." I gave her a blast out my solar plexus. We were having fun. Meg's husband wanted in and asked us to show him where he was open. I ran my hand up his body fields and told him I felt the solar plexus was strongest. The Aborigine-trained girl concurred. He said, "But I'm a good person, why isn't my heart chakra strongest?"

"I'm not certain goodness and chakras coincide but it could be interpreted that you still have to think about it. The solar plexus is associated with strong intellectual activity while the heart is considered more feeling," I replied. He seemed satisfied with that. The young woman had me march around the energy some more. I showed her how to change colors with intent. We were late for the next triad.

My next group included a woman from Puerto Rico who was attending because she had an ovarian cyst. She did not like the prospect of going under the knife. A small elf-like woman was kneeling before her, directing energy into her lower abdomen. I could see the elf didn't have the juice for what she was trying to accomplish, so I laid my hand on her shoulder and began to pump energy down her heart meridian. The look on her face was classic. Her name was Lisa Graves and she said, "Wow, what the hell are you doing?"

"I'm just feeding you. Take it and do what you know how to do. I use this stuff for breaking bricks. I can generate for hours. Go for it." She returned to her work and I continued to breathe energy into her while she directed it into the lady from Puerto Rico. That woman snapped to attention, her eyes rolled back in her head, and she went into orgasm. Meg and Barb came over to watch us at play while our victim vibrated. Blue light was running in little streams all up her body and over her face. It was like she was being electrocuted with microwatts.

Finally Lisa says, "I got it." I moved around the falling woman, guided her over to a massage table, and lifted her on to it. I ran my hands through her fields and she seemed to be burning very clean to me. I asked Lisa to check her out. Meg came over and did a pass, as did Barb. Barb adjusted the woman's hip. We all felt very pleased with ourselves. Lisa told me that she'd never worked with anyone that way before. I didn't tell her it was a first for me; I responded like old and knowing. Lisa and I became friends. I wandered off to talk with Barbara Allen and watch how she worked. She does a great wise woman and has a nice sense of humor.

When the seminar was over I was at the door talking with Sue from Chicago and the Australian-trained girl. Meg came over and said, "Dr. Morris, I have to apologize to you." I said, "For what?" She replied, "For what I said to you." I said, "Your response came from the heart and was absolutely correct for what and who you are. Think about it. No apology is necessary. I had a lovely time in your seminar." And I left with Lisa to see what kind of techniques she was willing to turn loose.

I bought Lisa dinner as she was dirt-poor, having scraped together every cent she had for this particular seminar. We went to my room and I had a beer. She being a healer told me she didn't drink. I showed her how to see energy in the mirror and breathe properly to generate more power. I took some of her healing energy and ran it through me using the internal witness to observe.

It was nice and pink and lit up all the meridians and organs. She knew her stuff. I showed her how to do a non-sexual exchange. She said, "When you do that, I see what looks like a demon in flames surrounding you, but it doesn't scare me. Why's that?"

"There's nothing to be afraid of," I replied. "It's tame now." She took off for home, but as she was going out the door Lisa turned and said, "You weren't kidding about being there to play, were you?" It seemed a heartfelt compliment. I have her work on my legs when I'm down that way. She lives in Charlestown, Indiana, and works in a health spa in Lexington. She is real good with ripped muscles and other mundane consequences of over-enthusiastic training. Someday I'd love to do a full split and lay my chest on the ground without screaming. It will take considerable stretching and bodywork to achieve that goal at my age, with my body.

The next day of the convention was Rubenfeld Synergy with Ilana Rubenfeld. She combines energy use with bodywork and psychotherapy and has her own school in New York City. She's world-class and a former Association for Humanistic Psychology president. I definitely wanted to observe her at work. Her day-long workshop was entitled "Healing the Mind-Body-Spirit Connection." It was attended by approximately 120 women and 30 men. She led us through some Feldenkrais-type exercises and eventually asked for a volunteer to get on her table. The session was being recorded.

A woman leaped from the crowd and Ilana started talking to her as she massaged her feet. I could see she was using intent but couldn't tell anything as her energy use was very subtle, with everything going into the woman on the table. Suddenly the woman began to babble the most horrific stories of sexual abuse and rape as a small child, beatings as a wife, divorce, remarriage, more abuse, harassment, on and on, one terrible event after another. If I had a client like her I would have been paralyzed. Ilana took each event and derived a lesson from it that led to the next event she might make a joke from. She subtly rebuilt this woman in one of the most virtuoso performances of the art of therapy

I've ever seen. It was astounding, the audience seldom made a sound, and the anger and sadness from the empathetic, primarily female group were palpable. Tears were streaming down my face. I could hardly breathe I was so shocked by her pain and their empathy. (There are many occasions when occult science is a painful disadvantage. It's referred to as compassion.) Ilana, like some sort of legendary pain-eating shaman, evoked memories with her touch, kneaded them out of the flesh, and discussed them into palatable lessons to avoid repeating. When she was finished she helped the laughing rag doll of a woman off the table. The woman was radiant, she was reborn. The atmosphere in the room did not bode well for men. I noticed there were about fifteen now.

She asked for another volunteer, and a young, athletic, beautiful woman with a withered leg climbed onto the table. Ilana started to rub her feet and relax her legs. The volunteer started to talk about her relations with men, and how hard it was to find a good one. Who would accept her? She was one of the last victims of polio. She had a sense of humor about her handicap or challenge. She described a dinner with the man she would like to marry and how he manipulated her and held back because of her leg. I turned to the woman sitting next to me, an attractive Ann Arbor type about my age in all handmade cotton clothing with thick grey hair to her thighs and gorgeous skin.

"I hope to hell she goes hunting," I whispered. She looked at me, tugged at her shawl, and grinned back. "So do I!" I felt a little better but the bad vibes for the masculine side were intense. I was working hard not to lose it. When Ilana finished with this volunteer, she whipped around and said, "Well, so much for women. I'd like to do a man now."

Nobody moved. No way. This group of female therapists was primed for blood. I think there were about five men left in the huge room. Silence was stretching when I found myself standing and moving toward the table. I had to experience this.

I climbed onto the table and introduced myself. She had me take off my jewelry and admired a dragon crystal neck chain made for my be Laura Butler, who specializes in fantasy designs. Ilana went to work on my feet, and the lady in cotton brought me her shawl to use as a pillow. I closed my eyes, went into no-mind, and turned my attention inward to see if I could catch any of her skills. She stretched my legs out and started a little relaxation massage when all of a sudden these nuclear bombs of energy started to flow up my meridians to explode behind my eyes. I was lost. She had me. I hoped nothing too gross would come out in front of this audience. I was semi-comatose when I heard her saying, "What's going on? How old are you?" I heard myself replying, "Five," in a small high voice. "Why are you crying?" she asks. "I'm being beaten by my Sunday School teacher," I wail. "She caught me eating the oatmeal paste and she's mad."

We then went into a three-way discussion with adult Glenn, little Glenny, and Ilana as interlocutor. We had a lot of fun and wrapped it up with me giving the little tyke words of wisdom like "Eat the goddamn oatmeal. It too will pass." When I got off the table she pressed her palms together and gave me a little bow. Hell, I'd give her a floor-knocker bow any time. That oatmeal incident could explain a lot of mistrust of authority. We did a little tai chi dance to the music and I escaped with my nasty, male-chauvinistic, androgynous self unrevealed. God knows what would have come out of me if she'd loosened up some other knot. It's a brave man that gets on her table in front of a national audience. You have no control at all. Rubenfeld Synergy. Kings of old would kill to have a seer like her work on them after a battle.

John Yono is a Chaldean Christian who owns a party store in South Lyon, Michigan. Meeting John is a bit like stepping into the pages of the fictional book *The Way of the Peaceful Warrior* by Dan Millman. Johnny is a boxer and self-taught madman. He follows the way of fire and can hit harder and faster from any direction than most professionals. There were no teachers who could handle him in the Detroit area, so he soon went his own way. When he was younger he used to train heavyweights for tough man contests. He's about 5'8" and weighs around 160. He fought his way out of the inner city and now trains by hunting and fishing around his store. He loves cars and has built one national championship hot rod. He is meticulous in running his store and raising his children. There is always some soup or wild game cooking on the gas grill in the back room for favored visitors. He keeps track of the gossip and politics of the neighborhood and the foibles of his neighbors. He knows everything worth knowing about all his customers. When they're down and out he provides credit and chow, and sends them on their way smiling. He's in his late thirties and looks twenty-three. His memory is phenomenal. He loved his mother and deeply grieved when she died; he visited with his father every week until the old man died, too. His father was from Iraq and made a place for his family in the wilds of Detroit. The old man had been very depressed since the death of his wife. He wouldn't leave the house. He was in mourning for over a year. The old man liked to fish but had never been lake fishing. Johnny and I rented a charter boat and took him out on Lake Michigan after salmon. We had a ball and the old man began to enjoy life again, but soon followed his beloved wife into the void.

I like to sit behind Johnny's deli counter and chew the fat while he supervises the teenagers who work for him. Occasionally I'll go to his house and we'll work out in his basement gym. After he gets done terrorizing me we'll take a sweat in his sauna. Usually we end the evening watching his hundreds of multi-colored wild fish from Lake Tanganyika in Africa swim around in their tanks. There's a big white male he calls Hatsumi because it hides so well and refuses to eat from his hand. John's a real human being. He's a martial arts friend. When one of my students wants to improve in boxing skills, I send them to Master Yono.

Leo Sebregst is head of the South African National Wu Shu Association. His dojo is a multi-storied building across from the police headquarters in Johannesburg. He has a farm in the Transvaal where some of the wildest kung fu training in the world is commonplace. He trains people of all races. As you walk up a hill in the high bush you see rising before you on the crest a Chinese-style wall. Leo and his students have built a temple fortress on top of a mountain. It's complete with a huge dragon's head entrance (you go in through the mouth) and bunkhouses overlooking the surrounding valleys. The view is spectacular. Leo says the idea of it came to him in a dream. He has made the dream reality. Nearby there is a climb up a brush-filled ravine that is done at night. One gets to acquaint oneself with scorpions, leopards, wild pigs, and other fun denizens of the farm. He has balance pole sparring arenas set up at different levels of difficulty and various other kung fu training devices to make the sides of the temple hill look like an obstacle course for the completely demented. I was flabbergasted. Kung fu students come from all over South Africa to train with this outspoken and talented man.

A colleague and hoshinroshiryu founder, Dr. Richard Grant, an economist at Witswatersrand University, invited me to be his guest in South Africa so I could see the country, meet Leo, and get an unbiased peek at the infamous situation. Now who would pass that up regardless of their political persuasion? I hopped a plane for Rio de Janiero and then took the southern route across the Atlantic. South Africa is well worth visiting. I loved it and can see why feelings concerning the political situation are so strongly held. (Rio, with its pickpockets, feral children, beautiful beaches, and people is another story concerning misguided government.)

SiGung (Grandfather) Sebregst's kwoon/dojo is brightly painted in traditional Chinese colors with smooth concrete floors and modern conveniences. He teaches in a gruff, fatherly manner and among martial artists I've observed is definitely in the grandmaster arena when it comes to control and movement. He's almost twenty years younger than most and so is just hitting his full powers. His hands are soft and cool but the skin feels a bit like a football, as he has used the traditional skin-toughening techniques of pounding sand, then gravel, and so forth. The sand is specially prepared with herbs to prevent infection, and a special tea is drunk to prevent blood clots. Eventually the skin is thick but smooth. The effect is quite different from the knuckle busting of karate.

We talked about some aspects of yin energy use, and Leo answered some questions that I'd never been able to find answers to among people whose English or experience was broad enough to respond. After we became comfortable with one another he asked me to demo for his students. I was a godan in hoshin, a sandan in ninjutsu, and a sifu in chi kung at this point and thought it would be fun to compare and contrast styles for a select group of eight or ten.

The evening demo was performed for well over a hundred of his upper-level students. I would demonstrate a technique and compare it to one from ninjutsu or kung fu. Then I'd answer questions. One long-haired young man asked me what drugs were preferred by ninjas. I told him to study homeopathic medicine and look into ginseng as a general anodyne. Then Leo demonstrated techniques that he perceived as parallel from the systems he taught. This went on for an hour or so, and then I was interviewed by the local martial arts magazine. An interesting night.

The interviewing reporter told me he was really surprised to find this interview and demo being conducted at Sebregst's, as Leo had often publicly stated and demonstrated in competitions his contempt for all the other martial artists in South Africa. (Leo has a little work to do around the concept of humility.) To have someone from another system actually giving a demo in his place was unheard of. I truly felt honored. Later Leo arranged for me to receive a teacher's license from the governing wu shu committee in case I decided to stay in South Africa. It became part of a collage I made of my martial adventures and hangs with my memorabilia.

A good friend once bought me a Christmas gift of an hour's therapeutic massage from a French masseuse who had been trained in Sri Lanka. She was very skilled and every now and then would lift her hands off me to measure or test my energy fields. She had never worked on a chi kung practitioner before. Not too many hang out in deepest darkest Lansing. So her curiosity was understandable. When she was finished I asked her if she had noticed anything strange that I should be careful about. She gave me a long thoughtful look and said, "Do you know you have a Buddha living inside you?" I laughed, "Yeah, he's eight hundred years old and doesn't know how to act. I have to take him everywhere but don't speak his language. It's a burden I have to bear. What would you do?"

"I don't know, Monsieur. I have never seen or heard of such a thing before." She isn't alone there.

The best student I ever had is an Ethiopian. His name is Toffesse Alemu. His father was a general and Toff grew up in Haille Selasse's household. He's a devout Coptic Christian and we've had many interesting discussions concerning Africa. He told me his grandfather had practiced many of the elements of hoshinjutsu and told him a true warrior had the soul of a great woman, spoke only from the heart, and breathed from the feet. He thought the old man was mad as a hatter.

Toff was raised with no concept of money. As part of the royal household, members of his family could walk into any business, select what they wanted, and the bill was sent to the palace. His father had him flying jets by the time he was fourteen. He has a Nilotic build and had never experienced prejudice until the Communists took over and his family fled to America. When he started his studies with me, he was in his mid-twenties, not terribly well coordinated, and his English was sub-high school. Being raised like a prince Toff had marvelous confidence and great mental discipline. He flunked every belt test at least twice as he worked his way up the ladder of hoshin, thus gaining deeper knowledge by continually returning to the basics with greater humility. Watching him struggle with the concepts through at least two languages taught me quite a bit about what can be communicated verbally and nonverbally. In a couple of years his physical and mental skills far surpassed my own. I have never been able to interest him in ninjutsu, and he regards me as his only sensei.

One of my other students who shall remain nameless belonged to the Klu Klux Klan (Hillsdale attracts conservatives of all stripes). He used to read to Toff from white supremacist literature. Here's a fool who thinks the mystic concept of "blood in the face" has something to do with race, lecturing an offshoot member of the oldest known royal bloodline in the Western world on white supremacy. Toff listened graciously, and then proceeded to advance far beyond this boob, who eventually drugged and drank himself out of college.

About a year into my second marriage I was lying in the bathtub alternating between reading a journal, meditating, and playing with my daughter's rubber duckies, when my wife Linda walked in nude with my grandfather's straight razor in her hand and sat on my chest. Now when a woman you love leaps into your bath with an open razor in her hand, you tend to be very still and pay attention. She wanted to shave my head, and since she had my arms pinned with her knees, I found it difficult to object. I also thought it was terribly funny. She proceeded to do it, humming softly all the while, and she only nicked me once.

The next day I went to work at the Dow Center and raised a few eyebrows. My colleague Dr. Kayne asked, "What's your wife going to say when she sees your new haircut?" I looked stern and replied, "The bitch will learn to love it!"

I still wear my hair shaved twelve years later. It doesn't have anything to do with kung fu or ninja commitment. I think Linda has a fixation on bikers or worse. It does give me an advantage when practicing throwing people by their hair.

Chapter Twelve

Screwing Up...
Higher Sexual Practice

IN 1986 I was asked to be an expert witness at the trial of a poor bastard accused of murdering another man by his former student/girlfriend/mistress who claimed she was his "ninja sex slave." You can imagine the uproar in Port Huron, Michigan. He wasn't a ninja and he didn't have a chance, although there seemed to my mind plenty of evidence of his innocence. He was just a not-too-bright tae kwan do teacher taking advantage of the ninja boom and couldn't keep his peanuts in his pants. He went to jail for a long time on hearsay and very sketchy evidence from a teenage girl and a flamboyant attorney waving *Original Ninja* magazine at the jury. His teenage wife was pregnant. His teenage sex-slave mistress was into drugs. During foggy walks in the riverside park, he told her about the *yakuza* (Japanese crime families) smuggling boatloads of dope in from Canada. The "ninja" had witnesses he was hundreds of miles away when the very public shotgun killing took place. The girl sex slave and a friend saw him speeding away from the scene in a car. The DA was up for re-election on a get-tough-with-criminals ticket.

The police sent five patrol cars, a SWAT team, and a helicopter to arrest the defendant. Ninjas with sex slaves are dangerous. He had *shinai* (bamboo training swords) in the trunk of his car and a

155

knoife (large Australian cutting tool) collection that wouldn't quit. Sexuality can create some interesting problems when martial arts are involved, particularly as an adjunct to enlightenment. It's not a good idea to screw up with your students. Save it for your friends or lovers.

In all my years of training in ninjutsu, sexual practice has never been a formal topic of discussion. Most of the instructors don't think in terms of sex therapy or sexual energy. As "warriors" they tend to be pretty macho and miss out on most of the fun stuff. Usually only the girls in the art know how to dance, which is fine by me. However, as a scholar of Taoism I have noticed that the Chinese students of sexology are a long way ahead of Masters and Johnson, and have been for at least a thousand years. If excellence in the pursuit of enjoyment includes spirituality in your sexuality, then you really have to face East for your inspiration. In hoshin we researched by comparative analysis where possible, as I like people to be informed concerning topics that are important to their happiness. In this section I'll discuss the psychological map and some physiological results of higher voltage, but if you want to check on the hard wiring and plumbing in the spirit house, check out the books I recommend in the bibliography and throughout these chapters.

To the common mind, sex and spirituality do not mix. (For that matter, neither do martial arts and spirituality seem a winning combination to most conventional thinkers!) Christian saints of the Roman Catholic version tend to be celibate, as do swamis. Tantrism contradicts this popular assumption as does most of history. You probably weren't taught much in junior high about Ben Franklin's girlfriends or Washington's and Jefferson's mistresses. Aside from the Nag Hammadi translations of the Dead Sea Scrolls, and the Gospel of St. Thomas, I don't recall ever being told about Jesus's seven female disciples. History is written by the winners or those who hold the power of censorship. If you want to get beyond the junior-high version of practically anything important about people, you have to do your own research and you have to know how to identify bias. Celibacy is a great concept for those who are ignorant concerning sex, or whose experience has been so negative or unattractive that doing without sex betters their lives. Finding people in the first category is not easy in this age of information and mass media. Those in the second group are on their own.

Celibacy can be a tool for increasing your awareness of your sexuality, and if male, retention of your sperm can enhance your energy, but the resulting increase in sensitivity translated to irritability in most adults is not a pretty sight. There are better ways and they are well documented if you know how to look. This chapter is provided to give you some hints, tools, and preventative measures while ensuring you have a better time than an ascetic. We're Americans. We're allowed to do this. Go for it. Crazy wisdom is for consenting adults.

An interpreter of esoteric traditions that I've come to trust, Georg Feurstein, is the author of *Yoga: The Technology of Ecstasy* and *Holy Madness: The Outer Limits of Religion and Morality.* Feurstein writes that Marpa (1012–1097, founder of the Kagyupa school of Vajrayana Buddhism, better known as Tibetan Tantrism) had eight tantric consorts in addition to his chief wife. (Moslems and Mormons are/were allowed four. Nine is a symbolic number to Buddhists.) Milarepa (1040–1143, the most famous of Marpa's students, considered the greatest Tibetan poet) was a folk hero as well as a weather magician. He liked to sing naked, as well as build towers and suffer Marpa's abuse. Milarepa is known to have initiated several of his female devotees. The *avadhuta* (Zen or "crazy wisdom" form of enlightenment) Drukpa Kunley (1455–1570) initiated more than five thousand women into the sexual secrets of tantrism. As the tantric techniques are similar to the Taoist, that may help to account for his longevity. He also was said to enjoy beer, humor, conflict, and poking fun at his monastic contemporaries and the governing authorities.

The avadhuta tradition or "crazy wisdom" is justified by its practitioners because from their viewpoint the general population needs a more drastic means of awakening to overcome its insensitivity, inability to shake material distraction, lack of compassion, and ignorance of the sacred order. "Shock" therapy is not only preferable but necessary, as the quiet example of the world-renouncing ascetic is not getting their attention. This insensitivity to subtle reality is often encouraged by authoritarian social institutions as a means to control members. Modern psychologists like Fritz Perls resemble the ancient avadhuta.

In the practice of clinical psychology, most self-destructive neurotic behavior comes out of warped sexuality, perverted religion, or parental abuse. Healing usually requires self-acceptance and self-forgiveness. Involvement of the abuser is not necessary to the process of forgiveness and acceptance. Perfectionism is the other major source of neuroses, related to and sometimes referred to as fear of failure. It can also develop into pronounced personality splits. The preferred cure is the realization at the deepest level of the strengths within your weaknesses, and acceptance and use of that knowledge. Many of us who grew up in the straight-laced fifties went through a bursting-out process during the sexual revolution of the sixties. Sexuality was never discussed except in awe and horror in the Morris household.

At the age of eighteen when I joined the army, after one year at Penn State studying philosophy, my father decided it was time to give me the words of wisdom to guide my sexual life. He came to my bedroom the night before I left for Basic Training and said, "Keep your mouth shut. Keep your nose clean. Don't go out with girls you are not introduced to!" I know he thought it was helpful. This is from a man with six children. Mom was equally forthcoming. Somewhere between storks and not-very-helpful biology texts there was a reality yet to be experienced, but they weren't giving a clue. It was typical of the time and of Fundamental Christianity. Why conservatives fear the awakening of their children must be connected to guilt, because ignorance is not bliss.

Given the record of sexual gurus in this country, I'll suggest that you're probably better off to experiment on your own or with the cooperation of a good friend and lover. You're not supposed to get too attached to the body. You might put a lot of so-called experts and professionals out of work if you really started to pay attention. The development of chi greatly alters your perspective concerning sex and increases the dangers as well as the pleasures. You would be foolish to abandon your critical intelligence to a teacher in this important area of learning.

Many of the women (and men) who develop an interest in the martial arts do so out of fear of men, fear of rape, and fear of physical abuse, which has not collapsed into the lethargic acceptance of domination, as they still aren't afraid or unwilling to learn to fight competently. Occasionally women are attracted to the spirituality within martial art, but find little of it in the men who train with them. They often seem to be receiving what they came to learn how to avoid. They may not handle pain well if it reminds them of other things. It is easy to drive such women from the dojo. It is easier to teach a woman who thinks it is fun to fight, or has at least been active in some physical sport like soccer, basketball, or best yet, dance, so she is used to pain. One should never confuse pain with joy, particularly your joy and their pain. Consider the rest of this chapter a guide to your own experimentation.

I had planned to write a long chapter with exercises and meditations, but after reading Margo Anand's *The Art of Sexual Ecstasy* (Tarcher) I was so impressed by most of her methodology that I'm only going to make a few comments and suggestions. One should read Douglas and Slinger's *Sexual Secrets* (Aurora) for a historical context as well as another viewpoint which supports and adds to what Ms. Anand has put in the public record. Mantak and Maneewan Chia's books concerning Taoist esoteric yoga and the cultivation of male and female sexuality (see bibliography) should also be read because they are the best internal researchers writing in English. These books will keep you busy and happy for quite a while, and with them you will probably avoid some of the dangers that I'll now describe which apply primarily to men, but not necessarily.

In kung fu some of the schools have names that can be translated as "Softening the Bone," "Shrinkage of Private Part," and "Beneficial Cessation of Desire." A corresponding metaphor in ninpo might be "Tiger Slaying Dragon Ryu." The tiger metaphor has to do with the female energy, learning to be more yin, using the energy channels that run up the front of the body. It is usually associated with negative or drawing energy. Men usually have to soften up considerably to even be aware of these meridians and the power that can move through them. I remember a Canadian student of ninjutsu pointing out to me that most of the Japanese senior instructors with their interests in art and dance struck him as being "rather limp-wristed." I pointed out that this was simply a cultural difference and there was no need to guard himself in the shower! I certainly wasn't going to bring up androgyny to him.

Gender-based behavior is largely socialized behavior and has little to do with biological sex, but a lot to do with how we think those of our own gender should act. It is the first part of the social self learned, and at a time when our judgment is least critical, making such behavioral choices a stable part of your personality by as early as the third year. Gender identification is learned personality and part of the structure of the social self and ego. It's part of what gets killed on the warrior path. Robert Bly and Gloria Steinem are pointing at a reflection.

Westerners tend to pay more attention to the strength that moves up the back, which is considered male or yang. Yang energy tends to be hot, whereas yin energy is cool. Yang energy is associated with the lower chakras and is considered dragon energy; its base color is red. Yin energy is associated with the upper chakras and is considered tiger energy. (It helps to remember that tigers are white in Tibet!) Yin lightens the energy in all the chakras as well as cools the internal organs. In the West we used to speak of being lion-hearted. It might be remembered that the Norse achieved Valhalla by being lifted from their deaths by the female Valkyries.

One might recall the folk wisdom pertaining to "being cool" or the description of someone sexy as "being hot." "Opposites attract" relates to hot women and cool men and usually to hot men and cool women. There may be a relationship between homeostasis and harmony. Similars seem to have the best long-term relationships, but difference may generate higher passion. I've seen descriptions of the colors and energy relating in different ways from what

I've just described, but this is how my personal experience leads me to share these appearances with you. Observe, experiment, and make your own conclusions.

One strengthens the energy in the body through deep belly breathing. The intestines serve as a coil to hold the energy as well as a pump to move it. Breathing techniques that move the intestines as well as fill the lungs are essential to higher energy as well as "higher sex" to use Anand's term. Once skill is developed in breathing, one usually notices that he or she spends an awful lot of time in the pursuit of sexual pleasure (pleasure being more interesting than simple reproduction) .

It seems to me that someone who learned these techniques when young enough to both enjoy and employ them would probably avoid most of the problems that are created when sexuality and spirituality are separated. Courtship and romance are the civilized equivalent of the hunt, and sexual conquest, the kill. It's probably the nicest way to get the hormones pumping. Marriage or acquiring a permanent helpmate can be regarded as the ultimate test, as the ramifications for the skilled hunter and huntress can affect generations. This may seem trite as an observation, but we tend to forget our animal natures when masked by the distractions of the polis. When we think about sex objectively, we also tend to forget that the other gender hunts, too. Marriage between equals is one of the higher forms of spiritual development as well as a reflective symbol used in human alchemy. The recognition of equal and different becoming the same is considered sacred and should be.

I don't pretend to understand women, but there is a Texas truism that has always made me laugh: "The thing that men keep forgetting about women is that if it weren't for procreation, there would be one hell of a bounty on them!" Being somewhat involved in the raising of three very different daughters and having grown up in families with traditions of working women, I like, to quote Bob Seger, "to watch her strut." Kali is the most feared manifestation of Shiva, who is also known as the kind one as well as the destroyer.

161

There are distinct differences between the sexes that may in some ways explain mating patterns as well as the value of androgyny. I refer to research on brain development and compartmentalization. The female corpus collosum permits significantly more energy to flow between segments of the brain, strongly suggesting that the bicameral brain is much more of a male problem than one for the female. The corpus collosum is seen by some psychologists as the seat of the Void. As a woman has greater access to her brain's storage capacity, she is more sensitive than a man. She is more alert to smell, touch, and sound. She has better hand-eye coordination. She sees better and is more skilled at reading and projecting the social cues of body language. She smiles more than men when she is not happy and is nicer to people she may not like—which could be considered a positive defense mechanism. She has a better memory for faces and character. These could all be considered side effects of having the right hemisphere of the brain better connected to its left side, which controls verbal expression and relationships. The intuitive is more in touch with communication skills. The mature female maintains closer, longer, and more confidential relationships than is typical of the male. She also seems to know when to cut her losses and split the blanket. All are strategic characteristics for a martial artist who values survival over conflict. To quote the fictional hard-boiled Detroit detective Amos Walker, "Sweet women lie."

It has been said about American men that maintaining one's lawn is more important than maintaining one's friendships. After the age of thirty the making of new friends is rare for men as most of our energy is put into "getting ahead." It is a sad commentary on life in modern industrialized civilization that the very pursuits that create a comfortable lifestyle for our families can blight personal development. Even successful women have not relaxed the pressure on men to succeed. Success is measured financially. If women are sex objects, then men are success objects. Most embrace the system with little consideration beyond their wallet. The emphasis on financial reward taints activities that were once regarded with respect. We are losing the concepts of husbandry, craftsmanship, friendship, and individual personal development.

One should really examine what it is to be a human being, what it takes to be happy. What goals are one's own and what have been imposed by the expectations of others? Where is this linear charge taking us? The famous Indian saint Yogananda found he did not have to go to the Himalaya (which he really wanted to do in his youth) because he achieved his heart's desire in his attic bedroom. The pursuit of money alone renders many young men marginal to our society and they are the primary source of crime and violence. Training in a no-competition and no-rules martial art provides friendship, respect, and challenges both physical and spiritual. Measuring others by their income was and still is considered a form of prostitution in my home. I've been rich and poor and at speeds that allowed me to watch the reactions of acquaintances to the rise and fall. Wealth is more fun than poverty but doesn't do much for character. That viewpoint is increasingly rare since Reaganism glorified image over substance beyond all historical precedent. Public power is sexy to some regardless of morality, and the media should pay more attention to the relationship than the act. Everybody screws. How you feel about it during and later is probably more important. I find the increasing sexual dissection of politicos funny, as the media should be delighted that some candidates who actually seem capable of love have been able to maintain relationships with intelligent, educated women, and have not alienated their children or beat them into submissive stereotypes.

Social interaction between the genders always relates to politics and wealth as well as biology. One may notice, if their biogenetic luck of the draw wasn't too good and their energy level not too high to begin with, that sex can be pretty draining. Hence all the warnings about preserving your seed and girding up your loins before battle. Both Chia and Stephen Chang (see bibliography) present a simple solution to this problem through manipulation of the perineum. There are Taoist myths of vampire queens who drained the life force of thousands of youths in order to attain

163

immortality. Harems maintained by males were not described in such negative terms, but it is strongly suggested that friendly sexual interchange with younger women is beneficial to sustaining one's youthful characteristics. What's good for the gander is probably good for the goose even in this day of voracious venereal disease. The French prefer that older women initiate younger men, which eliminates a great deal of male stupidity concerning how to treat women.

I remember reading an archaeology report of a fifth-century Scottish dig where the sewers of the castle rendered up thousands of little tied-off pieces of sheep intestine. With today's sexually transmitted diseases your protection has to be tougher than mere birth control. It is the friendly interchange that is important. This is exchange of valued energy and healing, loving commitment.

Sex is a waste of time, energy, and effort when partners are tired, aren't loving, enthusiastic, or skilled, or have a death wish. However, wasteful sex on the physical plane is better than no sex at all because one can still fool oneself into feeling loved. Loving touch is remarkably therapeutic. Let us not in our pursuit of spiritual purity forget biological reality. Creating a child is a twenty-year responsibility and should not be treated lightly. I've seen parents who don't have the tools to raise a cat, let alone a viable child. Passing on a venereal disease, like date rape, is not a loving act. Bacterial-based disease does seem to be eradicated by the strengthened immune system. Stephen Chang suggests that high levels of chi prevent venereal disease. My experience is chi only slows down viral-based disease. Viruses are complex and tricky. Flu, herpes, chlamydia, and AIDS are viral. I've no interest in personally testing Dr. Chang's hypothesis, but I'll bet he's wrong. I've had flu two or three times since going through the kundalini and had the opportunity to educate a young friend concerning the spread of chlamydia, which is hard to detect in its early stages in the male, as it is a mild itching in the urethra similar to what you get from too much coffee.

We humans are the sexiest of the primates as well as the most successful in exploiting our environment through the tools and masks of culture. Unlike our less erect cousins, a female human being is always sexually accessible, even during pregnancy and nursing when she is more difficult to impregnate (something of an advantage when you'd like to keep a man about the house or cave). The male of the species has not only the longest but the thickest erect penis of all the 192 species of primates. The human is capable of greater variation, intricacy, and duration than any other animal. Testosterone, the aggression and dominance hormone, is also the sex hormone in both men and women. Testosterone is produced and controlled by the adrenal gland, which also plays a major role in stress management, the martial arts, and the pursuit of enlightenment. Men have twenty times the level of this powerful hormone in their bodies and brains than women, which when combined with the adrenals may account for a certain narrowness of focus. The jokes about women being hormone-driven are probably projective slander.

All the jokes about fallen gurus have in the root the simple equation that love and sex are similar and someone who is highly evolved is also highly sexed. It is how the sexual energy is applied that creates the definition—healing, prophecy, charisma, power-seeking, creativity, and breaking bones all flow from the same source. Higher sex requires sublimating the orgasm as well as exchanging energy with the lover. If one is skilled in the control of energy, penetration is not required to give a loved one orgasmic, loving, balancing, or healing energy. If coitus is involved, the male freezes the moment before ejaculation and then reverses the muscle spasms to pull the semen and sperm back into himself while projecting his energy into what is known as the G spot in the female. Or he could be drawing energy, depending on what the participants are trying to accomplish and their degree of skill. This takes a little practice and control, but it is fun to learn how to do. It requires attentiveness as well as considerable slowing down to capture the moment, because you will want to repeat the experience at will. Testicular kung fu or ovarian kung fu is considered one of the identifying skills of a Taoist master of the martial arts. I found learning it more engaging than the sumo technique of drawing one's testicles up into the body. Fear will do that for me, and faster. I know how to use my adrenal glands.

Penetration is not necessary to exchange energy nor is gender necessarily relevant. Knowing how to "work" your energy or chi or aura is. Two people can have a lot of fun trying to make it work, trying to make their microcosmic orbits link up. The exchange benefits both participants, if both give freely and with respect, as both are strengthened as well as harmonized. Yin to yang, yang to yin. The *yab yum* position (couple sits facing in meditation) in Tantric Tibetan lore is probably the most efficacious for this exchange. The tongue and the genitals might be considered the equivalents of male and female plugs for the connecting of the current. The spirit is bioelectrical in nature. This position works best cross-sex when you are relaxed but focused. Back to back is valid same-sex. Nurses trained in therapeutic touch make energy exchanges over considerable distances, as do tai chi and chi kung masters and some very high-level ninjas. It's all similar.

Respect, play, and healing are important parts of the formula. A woman should learn the positions known as *the secrets of the plain girl* (sexual healing techniques) and master the *big draw* (life force manipulation). A man at the very least should master *nine little heaven* (prolonged orgasm techniques) and *the million dollar spot* (sperm flow retention point) described by Stephen Chang. These are discussed in *Sexual Secrets* and *The Tao of Sexology.* Recently published research in the *Journal of Sex and Marital Therapy* indicates strongly that women who climax before or with their partners are happier than those who climax after their partners. Today men and women of college age and intelligence want a sexual partner with some experience. What they prefer is that their dates be potential mates and that there is emotional attachment with the involvement. Sexual relationships are preferred when there is more depth than simple mutual masturbation and more to share than simple belly rubbing. Passion far exceeds competence.

When chi is involved, the lover merges with the beloved as intent or feelings penetrate with both physical touch and tasting flowing together in their energy fields. In the beginning it is the soft feather touch of movement in the air above the beloved, and in the end it is stroking wafts of energy massaging the cellular structure of the pleasure centers of your beloved's brain, which can be reached by going down the meridians. The practitioners of non-contact therapeutic touch and tantric yoga and the esoteric martial artist have similar energy. The difference is in power, not perception. A lover of a physical art is no less a lover than a poet or a scientist and may have some surprising sensitivities not often explored by most people. I no longer can count the people who have been surprised by this knowledge, but were quickly able to take advantage of the benefits.

Now, the warnings for the males in my reading audience. Remember what I said earlier about microwattage increasing as your power increases. If your partner is on a lower wavelength or doesn't have much energy due to lack of physical conditioning or inattention, you will burn her, particularly if you don't bring her to orgasm, or she does not know how to do the "big draw." Women do not appreciate scorched vaginas. Neither do they enjoy migraines, barfing, and being wired out if you can't harmonize your energy to hers. If you don't figure out how to cool your tool you won't be invited back. On the other hand (decidedly left), the ones who do know about full-body, spirit-merging, blissful orgasms of indefinite time period tend to enjoy your attentions and reciprocate. Sometimes they send their friends around to enjoy something really different. I have had sexual partners faint both when dancing and making love; I'm not sure what to make of that other than circuit overload, incipient epilepsy, or good luck. They seemed to regard it as a surprising side effect of ecstasy. It has never happened to me. A prophylactic does not block energy exchange or in any way reduce ecstasy, in my opinion. These days it may even increase your pleasure if you don't know your friend's sexual history.

If sex wasn't much fun for you, or your experiences were primarily negative, as you draw the energy upward away from the genitals to feed the brain, you may find you lose all interest in what goes on below. Some schools of thought consider this a blessing. You may find you are now impotent. The chi-related impotence has two causes. Sex, being primarily negative for you, is no longer a driving force in your life. In other words, clarity of thought is more important to you than a hard-on. The other reason is you are not in love. The spirit does not lie. You just can't get it up when you don't care. Promiscuity falls by the wayside. Your marriage might too. As your mind and genitals are now connected, spontaneous erections will be a thing of the past. You might have to work harder on your foreplay (it's the dreaded "softening the bone"). The penis functions just fine, only slower. Some of the sisters inform me a little slowness is appreciated.

There are more than a few warnings in the Taoist literature recommending that a man should be certain of his own skill in generating chi as well as preserving his seed before initiating his female partner, as women are much better at all of this than men are. It has been my experience that if a girl or woman learns how to run the orbit she will be much more powerful both physically and sexually than most men. Being able to join and exchange your energy is the true meaning of soul mates. I won't even try to describe how wonderful that can be and how wrenching and horrible to lose it.

If you are overly rigorous in your pursuit of enlightenment and/or accidentally gain bliss by blowtorch before your body has been properly prepared, your pain and terror will probably forestall all sexual interest and women will be regarded from the Pauline or demonic perspective. It's no fun to be blinded in the desert. Every time you get an erection you tend to fall to your knees and throw up from the intense migraine caused by the energy movement to the skull, which has not been properly prepared to handle the raw, hot, and dry male reproductive voltage. In fact, St. Paul's complaints of symptoms sound remarkably like chi sickness. He also exhibited extraordinary abilities of self-healing, as he sustained substantial beatings and stonings during his ministry. Unlike Jesus, he didn't have much time for the fairer sex. He didn't make friends easily as he took his religion very personally. He was a rabble-rousing ranter and bad-tempered when he called himself Saul. I'll wager that one of the disciples that Saul had stoned to death managed to transfer some chi into him. Once in, it starts working its way to the top and the stronger spirit wins. It doesn't take long.

There are some schools of Magic in both Eastern and Western traditions that purely hate women. Women are to be treated as wicked animal distraction and regarded as demons. It's easily understood. Here's a perfectionist, been saving up his sperm for many years. Responsible for training young monks. He can read emotions. He can feel the inside of his liver. He's pure as the driven snow until the hot little tart that serves his food mentally whacks him in the pineal gland and starts providing all kinds of distractions that the founding fathers claim lead to damnation. He doesn't have any defenses; it's not part of his training. Monks don't get to spend much time around women until they've got a fair chance of fighting them off. Now, if this happens often enough, the scholars are going to get together to save the recruits from the horrors of losing their seed, or getting married and dropping out. They'll figure out "How to Have Power Over Women." If they're of the demon-regarding school, there's always exorcism or death.

You ever notice it's almost always the girls who get possessed or burned at the stake? Fear and intolerance quickly become institutionalized in stable societies. Women in many parts of Asia are treated only slightly better than a Doberman pinscher. When Drukpa Kunley initiated five thousand women he was a living Buddha. He was making a statement about human rights, women as spiritual vessels, guaranteeing the knowledge would be passed on to children, and probably having some fun too. Jokes about him are still told in Tibet today. He seems like a Holy Till Ullenspiegel. In Tibetan tantrism every male deity has a female consort who to an outsider would appear to be exceptionally bad news. Janusian females. Read up on Kali. Goddess worship can be pretty high-risk. Jesus liked to exchange footwashing. Kinesiology is another easy way to exchange energy.

169

Sexual energy is the primary tool of transmission by a tantric master or mistress. The spirit is not only energy but intent. Intentionality is a direction by definition. Knowledge to some extent can be transferred; at least feeling can. Powerful people's energy fields extend quite a distance from their bodies, and the more unrefined spirit begins to evolve simply through contact with their fields. When an energy master gives you his or her energy, it will change you. If you have not already opened yourself, the process will begin with or without your acceptance. It will just take much longer if you're not an active participant. Your spirit learns from her spirit. I describe some interchanges in the chapter "Exchanges with Interesting People."

In the martial arts we refer to this as "the stronger spirit wins." The process is more than behavioral monkey see, monkey do. It's a privilege to be beaten by a master. Energy has emotional content. It's another reason why happily married people begin to look and act alike. I once had a girl tell me that all the godan and above in the Togakure Ryu were "as alike as peas in a pod" in their attitudes. We all seem pretty different to me, but then I don't have her perspective. Being a yondan at the time, I would like to think she was reacting to the calm acceptance of others, the gentleness, or the intensity. Training as a hobbyist I'm not around that much. I usually only attend a seminar or two a year and have never studied under one particular teacher for any length of time. I do know that for the most part many of them do not seem tantric, nor shamanic, nor biologically enlightened. The higher energy is not always there. Taijutsu yes; the Void not yet. Only Hatsumi and one or two others continuously manifest, and as we're talking about a handful out of a hundred and fifty, I'd say the system is remarkably effective. After all, what is the ratio of enlightenment in the general public, or for that matter in our institutions that are designated for that particular project? I had a Catholic priest friend tell me one time that he liked vacationing at the monasteries because he felt the odds were about one in ten thousand there of meeting someone who was enlightened, as opposed to one in a million in the general population. He's still looking for light in all the wrong places. Even Merton went East.

If your spirit is weak or untrained, you are a sitting duck for anyone with a stronger spirit who has designs on you and even a rudimentary skill at energy manipulation. Or worse yet, someone who drains your energy and is incapable of generating their own. They're usually unaware that their negative mindset affects their energy and affects those with whom they interact. They're not vampires, they're just lost. I once had this verified by a woman I worked with who taught me a lot through sharing her experience and doing things to me that she'd think up.

In casual conversation about her neurotic boyfriend, she once laughed, "I used the Big Draw on him and really drained him. He nearly passed out. He didn't like it one bit!" She could lay two fingers on your hand with a gentle swirling movement and you could feel her move energy anywhere in your body. She could make you smile or laugh at twenty feet. (He didn't catch on and he didn't improve. They didn't get married.)

The major meridian of the heart which also connects into the brain and the genitals gets involved with sex. There is a story about William James under the influence of an anodyne asking the spirit of the drug the reason for psychological suffering. In the morning he found he had written:

> "Higamous, hogamous
> Woman is Monogamous
> Hogamous, Higamous
> Man is Polygamous."

He was not impressed, but from an anthropological perspective I've always thought it rather profound. Some biographers claim it was laughing gas and others mescaline.

Sex is still sex regardless of the intent, and all that wonderful creative energy is expressed in its most fundamental and biological power. Those skilled in chi kung simply draw off the energy at its rawest source and use it for transcendence rather than reproduction.

171

Tantric practice is also supposed to be a powerful method for birth control as it operates on two levels: preserving the seed and drawing off the little swimmers' energy in case any escape. The ignorant simply follow their biological and socially reinforced proclivity. The results are sometimes the same. Make love, not war.

There is a pretty strong rumor that one of the Tibetan tantric masters at Naropa who was a teacher of crazy wisdom confused sex and gender with androgyny and infected quite a few of his followers with HIV. Many are now dying of AIDS. He may have just about wiped out a major portion of the school. Good intention does not kill viruses. Safe sex avoids the disease as well as the issue. Being able to discriminate between fantasy and reality, I can't really recommend abstinence. Chinese medicine is no more infallible than our Western traditions but still has a great deal more to offer in knowledge of the bioelectric. Viruses are a domestic problem.

Chapter Thirteen

Mirror, Mirror . . . Seeing through a Glass Darkly

IN MAGICAL, RELIGIOUS, and occult practice, cryptic references are often made to mirrors. Folklore, superstition, and myths from many cultures mention the use of mirrors and not just for scrying. Lao's mirror reflected the mind and its thoughts. Merlin's mirror informed him of treason, secret plots, and other dangers to Arthur's kingdom. Vulcan's mirror showed the past, present, and future. Tezcatlipoca spoke to his Aztec supplicants as the Lord of the Smoking Mirror, and his mirror had the property of continually bringing faces to its dark surface as if seen through smoke. Practitioners of Zen refer to "polishing the mirror" as their actions are a reflection of the state of their souls. Ninjas do *kyojutsu* (weird air combat skills to subdue the demons).

Vampires and yidam cast no reflection and their shadows are thinner and lighter. (No self?) Many so-called primitive societies believe reflections, like shadows, are projections of the soul and avoid gazing into water or having their photographs taken as it may endanger their spirit. American Indian shamans often practice "face-dancing" in a mirror to demonstrate their degree of enlightenment. St. Paul looks "through a glass, darkly," and Aleister Crowley gives specific mirror-building directions to catch all the subtle nuances of the experience of reflection. There is more going on here; the word itself, reflection—illusion—deep thought, has many elusive meanings.

It seems to me that much smoke must reflect some fire. "Darkly" is the key to the experience. Usually when you look in a mirror, it's well lit. Light washes out what you are trying to see unless you are schizophrenic or under the influence of a hallucinogen. Drugs are not necessary but good night vision and control of your breath are. I discovered this on my own, but I've run into ninjas who have face-danced with teachers of shamanism. Brugh Joy makes the usual cryptic reference to mirrors in his book *Joy's Way*. If you were working a large group in a ballroom with mirrored walls, dim lights, and meditative music to increase the feelings of relaxation, what you might start to get in the mirrors after everyone was suitably relaxed would be well worth the creative energy necessary to be surprised again. My editor tells me this isn't real clear. Just do it. It has to be experienced.

The kundalini experience is not requisite to some of the phenomena I'll describe, but I'm fairly certain that it relates to some of the more bizarre aspects. First let me state strongly that this can be a very scary experience, and you will be much farther ahead if you've developed your powers of positive thinking, because what you get in the mirror is a reflection of your most basic self. The workings of the id are not always pretty nor do they always fit normal consensual reality.

My first mystical experience with a mirror was when I was stationed in Germany with the Third Medical Battalion. I was on guard duty, and during my off shift I set up a small mirror with a candle behind me and went into a meditative trance. Tolstoi describes a similar use for scrying with mirrors in *War and Peace*. I contemplated my girlfriend who was attending Northwestern University. In the mirror I saw her sitting in a large room with burnt-umber furniture and she was weeping. I wrote her a letter and she responded that she had just broken up with someone she'd been dating there and the room I described was the student lounge in her dormitory.

That was thirty-some years ago, and I never tried that one again, as wisdom has taught me it is better not to check into the private affairs of your lady loves. A voyeur's life is not necessarily made happier by his curiosity. What I'll describe next seems to be much easier to replicate, as it deals with self-revelation. Here's the recipe; the results have to do with how well you cook.

Set up a mirror in a darkened room. Provide enough light to see yourself faintly. Begin skin breathing, or pushing your energy out from your body. (This will work better if you meditate for a while and wait for your eyes to adjust to the dark.) Watch the mirror with minimal blinking and no expectation. Wait for whatever appears or scarier yet, disappears. Be as relaxed as possible and try to hold onto no particular train of thought. Let your normal consciousness become quiet so that your subconscious can more easily emerge. And just like Jesus in the Garden of Gethsemane, your face might change. Sometimes it's helpful to put a candle to one side (Musashi recommends the right), as the flickering makes you work harder to see subtle differences and the flame will bend as you begin to increase your energy. That's all it takes. A quiet mind, no expectations. You don't have to invoke the demon gods or sacrifice your children or suck anyone's blood to disappear in a mirror. (I showed Suzanne Carlson's father how to do this one night in London and he was able to get it in a couple of minutes with no prior experience. He now entertains his friends this way at cocktail parties. His wife has not forgiven me.)

If you've been meditating sufficiently to alter your body's electrochemical system and have become pretty good at stilling your ego, you may just fade right out. No reflection. In primitive societies this particular genetic proclivity toward night moves and skill is of great service to hunters, scouts, spies, and the righteous who have to flee and hide in the night.

I've tried this on different "wavelengths" and received interesting insights. When one practices chi kung or breath control as part of their meditative agenda it activates the parasympathetic nervous system and enhances the body's immune system. One of the effects of this is increased resistance to disease, and it is perhaps also the cause of a major change in the electrical fields that surround the body. In folklore this may be referred to as the aura or "vibrations." The trick to seeing it is being relaxed and using your night vision in the daytime which requires dilating the pupils, which also takes you slightly out of 20/20. Many people have noticed the glow around others, but as no one talks about it in terms of utility it soon becomes a part of our perceptual world we choose to ignore. (I discuss this in more detail in the chapter on aura seeing and feeling.) After all, the visual mechanisms of the brain have enough to do processing upside-down to right side up, as well as sidedness. (The way our optic nerves operate may have something to do with when we were fishlike, because as an adaptation to arboreal binocularism it seems awfully inefficient to me. A good physical anthropologist could probably give a more detailed explanation, but take it for granted the eye/brain link-up has some amazing filters to information-processing.) If one is rigid, no new information need apply. The rule "we hear what we want to hear" also applies to the unmindful observer in that "we see what we're supposed to see." When your mind is open you may see some things you are not supposed to see, or at the very least have forgotten or never learned how to see. The angling in ninjutsu and a few other arts takes advantage of a little-known blind spot in our eyes. Study on this.

The animal or biological aspects of human beings are more potent than the learned personality, but this unrecognized shadowy intelligence hides in the body's electric fields—probably from the days of toilet training when the young human being begins to be truly socialized. However, the id is with you, grown up and hopefully toilet trained, as this aspect of yourself has been observing your situation for all the years of your particular existence. It is still a child regardless of age, represents itself with icons, and is moral to a mythical degree. It is also a force of nature and thus recognizes its duality. When it shows you one side, like Janus or the Hindu gods, it also shows you the other. Joy is balanced by regret.

When I described the kundalini experience, I mentioned the unwinding of one's memory. I had an experience that might be analogous to Vulcan's mirror and which I hypothesize as genetic memory. I was "face dancing" in deep meditation one night but instead of the usual holographic shifts I began to see very clear faces and upper bodies superimposed one over the other: mostly male figures, a few females, some with long hair, some short, some bearded, some not, some heavily muscled, some clothed, some naked. As the faces changed and time passed (it seemed to go on for quite a while), the brows and chins became heavier until it seemed a parade of knuckle-walkers. Nobody was old; they all seemed to be in pretty good shape if a mite intense of aspect. It might be explained as genetic memory of one's forebears contained in the DNA/RNA, as all these figures were relatively young, of child-bearing age. It might be a confirmation of Nietzche's plagiarism of the wheel of dharma in that we keep coming back until we get it right. If so, I've been on this ride for an awfully long time. If there's such a thing as an old spirit, mine is decrepit. Some of those knuckle-walkers looked like neanderthals. What I'll describe next I perceive as more ordinary and have been able to demonstrate to students, friends, and (usually a mistake) lovers. Same process, different intent, different result. I've shown numerous people how to erase themselves in the mirror. A strange side effect of this for which I've no real explanation (a problem of being self-taught) is that sometimes the people I'm showing say that not only does the image fade out of the mirror but the person being reflected disappears as well. This could definitely put a damper on a romantic candle-lit dinner. I don't recommend it as a way to win friends and influence people; however, I suspect it has something to do with the fields occulting the light in some way because from my viewpoint only the mirror image fades. Sometimes when I'm doing this with a friend they will describe not being able to see themselves or me, but I still see them in infrared. We're experimenting with different light frequencies now. I think it is a camouflage adaptation for the more nocturnal primate. Ninjas are sometimes referred to as shadow warriors, and this cloaking effect might add another level to that description. "Shadow warrior" can also be interpreted as one who engages the darker side of one's self, as well as indicating a preference for engaging in battle in what lesser men and women would consider handicapped conditions. I have often trained in a darkened ninja dojo.

Sometimes when you observe this strange phenomena in mirrors you see the body surrounded by what appears to be colored flame, somewhat like the pictures in Tibetan icons. Sometimes you get faces that you can be pretty sure aren't you. Different sex, different age, different race, different species. And most interesting, if you focus from a particular chakra you may get the appropriate archetype. Depending on your propensity for positive thought as well as ferocity, you may not be too pleased at meeting your motivating demon and shadow self.

When sparring or engaged with particular martial artists able to project their spirit or who have acquired martial spirit guides, what you see coming out of the night at you besides their weapons and fists can definitely be a shock to the system. The person being attacked will feel regardless of whether he or she can "see." A spirit warrior can project this image before him or her. The image is either the archetype, or something that scared the opponent as a child. I rather fancied projecting the crypt keeper from the old horror comics that were banned, you may remember the one with the melting eyeball. I gave him up when friends started avoiding me. The archetypes that come up are often different variations of the trickster. I've seen Japanese *tengu,* which correspond to the Hopi horned god. When face dancing with someone of American Indian extraction, the *tulpu* (Tibetan for living apparition) are related to Indian mythology. Egyptian animal heads, particularly bird heads, seem to be common; it probably relates back to totem poles in some way that has been lost from the oral tradition. (The inner energy deities' archetypal nature could be represented hierarchically on a raised pole or phallus.) One of my students of Celtic extraction can project a great-looking tree king rather like Huon of the Horn complete with antlers, and she fades out real well too. For those who prefer Western "magick" I once got on the wavelength of a rather Elizabethan-looking gentleman who resembled a painting of John Dee, so if these are indeed spirits or spirit guides, some of the old-time European practitioners seemed to have escaped the wheel of return. I have had students project spirits wearing war masks. I haven't the faintest clue, except the masks resemble Tlingit artifacts. It's evident to me that these rather odd side effects could be easily exploited by a priesthood concerned with dominance and power.

I tend to regard with deep suspicion those who pursue Mesoamerican shamanism. Let us not forget all those virgin sacrifices (fear is a great source of energy as is innocence), and the members of winning basketball teams that got to meet their maker as a reward for their skill (so is religious exultation).

Under difficult light conditions a mirror or darkened window allows one to see projections. The mirror trick may also serve as a diagnostic device for seeing someone's motives or intention when you walk him or her by a mirror when it's dark. What you see may lead you to change your mind, but then again, fear no evil. Forewarned is forearmed. The dark is and can be your friend.

When Jesus meditated in the Garden and his face changed to that of one of the prophets, it might have been an example of channeling or the manifestation of a spirit guide. When describing the kundalini experience in chapter three, I mentioned my reservations toward channeling. However, prejudice aside, I seem to have acquired some curious Oriental fellow travelers that don't fit my preconceptions very well. When I project onto the mirror while doing deep belly breathing, I often get an old, wispy-looking Chinese who resembles pictures I've seen of the mythic Yellow Emperor. He comes through quite clearly and I've shown him to many of my friends who have esoteric interests. I've always liked Chinese art and poetry in translation, and the basic principles of kung fu make sense to me, as do the refinements of ninjutsu. Somehow, I feel very comfortable with this odd spirit (odd for a white preacher's kid from Pennsylvania). He usually floats slightly to the left in front of me.

When I hold my shoulders back with my head high while using a sustained exhale, my reflection becomes greenish and through me comes a fattish, shaven-pate Oriental who looks a lot like statues I've seen of Kobo Daishi, who I understand was the founder of Shingon Buddhism in Japan. He may have caught my train at Koya-san. This one is dressed as a Japanese and comes in two versions, middle-aged and about twenty-five: both feel the same. There are also three samurai types with ornate hairdos that seem to be close associates of the fat one. Once I got a *Kuan Yu* lookalike (Chinese war deity for shamans and artists). The more androgynous, shape changing beauty of Kuan Yin has eluded my search. I have no idea why these "people" are hanging out with me. I certainly don't live anything like a consecrated life. I've consciously avoided learning Japanese and Chinese to the embarrassment of my friends who feel learning the language is important to the study of ninpo. For them it is: for me, I'm a little worried that if I learn their language the spirits may learn mine, and if I were to start babbling in Enochian (the language spoken by angels, according to the Golden Dawn Society) while working with a bunch of managers, they might just throw a net over me. Channeling an ancient Oriental wouldn't add much to my credibility with the conservative organizations that hire my services. I think I'll wait, continue to be distant but interested, and work on my telepathy. I suspect I'm not unique.

The ancient Taoists said the number and type of spirits one acquired were reflections of his or her perception and power, as like attracts like. As I've seen little to indicate a Western slant to these apparitions, I reluctantly reject the concept of it all being genetic. It could be learned or worse yet acquired. If I had my druthers I'd rather bring through Falstaff or even John Wesley, who I would understand even though he wouldn't be much fun. I've always admired Ben Franklin.

There does seem to be an exchange of information that takes place on a feeling level between me and these disembodied playmates. As I said, I enjoy Oriental art, friendship, music, and food. There is definitely a sensual connection and appreciation of aesthetics not acquired at high school, college, or graduate school. I often know how to use ancient religious articles in nonordinary ways and understand the hidden meaning in rituals and paintings. It's very hard to verbalize. But I suppose it has something to do with how Tibetans identify a reincarnation. I'd like to observe that process. John White informs me that Eastern reincarnations are becoming quite common in the West and he links it to the Tibetan diaspora. I've had friends who thought the Hippie movement was an Indian ghost dance. I don't know. It appears heaven can wait.

As time passes, the energy of a particular spirit manifestation seems to merge with my own and the others. It becomes harder to draw out as a separate entity from yourself, but with a little mirror practice you can use the reflection as a feedback device as to whether you're able to sustain a particular attitude in depth. As you lose the mood, the spirit fades. As it/he/she becomes more in tune with your reality, it becomes more a part of you—thus spirit guides. There are situations where subtle suggestions from another realm of experience can be useful, particularly when it comes to fighting for your life or the situation has decayed to include fighting for your family. It is this heartfelt plea for survival to which the hormones respond, summoning the archetype, and it is only with total openness not demand for power that one gets to use the subconscious or spirit to solve the problem. The Muses are similar.

I have had "the fighting spirit" respond to an insult, and it was pretty funny to me if terrifying to the person who catalyzed it. It occasionally over-reacts or reacts in a way more appropriate to a less sophisticated society. I suspect that is why Sun Tzu suggests that the wise man will sometimes ignore the admonition of the spirit. These boys didn't have to contend with modern police methods. The violent spirits are triggered by the adrenals. They are easiest to see and feel. You don't waste this on what tie to select unless your guiding spirit is into fashion.

Chapter Fourteen

Dreams and Dreamers

REAMWORK IS AN esoteric area that has attracted scientific analysis in the last decade. There has been considerable research into lucid dreaming, where the dreamer takes control of the events in the dream or at least is aware of the fact he or she is dreaming. Psychologists have set up sleep labs to study student sleep patterns and have done quite a bit of physiological measurement in the last few years. The mystery is fading. The Winter 1992 (#22) issue of *Gnosis*, a magazine for Western esoteric traditions, devoted almost all of its articles to the use and understanding of dreams. Both Freud and Jung did extensive work with dream analysis and found a valuable resource.

The Sufis use dreams as part of their training, and many of the Christian and Judaic prophets used the content of their dreams to show their relationship to Jehovah. The Roman God-Emperor Claudius recorded dreams he thought were important, as well as his family's historical and profitable relationship with the water sprite Egeria. Roger Bacon, one of the founders of the Royal Academy of England, expressed an interest in dreams, as did his contemporary, the magician John Dee. Brugh Joy puts a great deal of emphasis on the interpretation of dreams. There's a long history of interest and research into what happens to the mind when we sleep.

The ninjas have techniques for the active use of dreams, and some have the ability to communicate in and with dreams across great distances. I have had both Hatsumi and Stephen Hayes convey messages to me in dreams. In both cases it was something I already knew how to do, so I incurred no giri. Dreamwork for the purpose of combat is a little different. It can be quite fun to send a nightmare to an enemy, depending on your skill in understanding his or her fears. Of course, you must study to be able to do this. It requires endurance on the part of your friends if they accidentally share your attempts to master Dreamtime.

On the next few pages, I'll lay out some basic ideas, convey some cautionary tales as warnings, and then leave it up to you. Dreamwork and creative meditation tap into similar areas of the brain. As even animals dream, which any dog or cat owner can observe, the area is obviously not the higher cortex. Dreaming can be considered a primitive function. Most psychologically healthy people do not remember their dreams as they are not warnings but simply entertainment for the mind while the body is sleeping. Dream content normally flows out of the four Fs of survival: feeding, fleeing, fighting, and sex. If a dream becomes a repeater, that is usually a sign that the spirit or body would like to get the social self's attention. Once the social self recognizes the problem, the dream goes away.

Before my first wife divorced me I used to have a recurring dream of wandering around a large, empty house with rotting floors. My companion in the house was a small, black, yappy bitch dog that attacked me every time I'd start to crash through one of the rotting spots. Disconcerting to say the least. Considering that she divorced me in the midst of the struggle to get the Ph.D., the dream content seems obvious. Hindsight is like that. At the time I made the mistake of describing the dream to her. She saw the implications where I did not. She was pissed. She was a psychological anthropologist and had read a lot of Freud. Freud felt that one of the major functions of dreams was to adaptively connect emotions to events. Dreams of this sort usually don't require a great deal of introspection if you're in touch with your feelings. (I wasn't at that time, or at least had trained myself as a medic to ignore most feelings, not wishing to be "sensitive.") Once the divorce was final, the dream went where all warnings that are heeded retire to.

The research on Rapid Eye Movement or REM sleep indicates that we usually dream a number of times in the course of the night. Lucid dreaming studies show that we can program ourselves to dream about particular topics by self-suggestion before dropping off.

Dreamwork times that are most effective seem to be just before going to sleep or just as you are waking up. When you realize you are beginning to dream, rather than just watch the story, raise up your hands and get into the situation just as an actor gets into his or her part. The entertainment hypothesis is supported by the fact that when I was a child most people seemed to dream in black and white, like the movies and television. (I've always dreamed in color.) I can't tell you how long it has been since anyone told me their dreams weren't in color. Taking an active part in your dream life is one way to train the imagination.

My son Shawn informs me he likes to edit outcomes as he goes, and if the dream starts to move in a direction he perceives as unpleasant he gets busy and changes it to his liking. He also tells me it is hard to get out of these dreams when you are interacting and something happens outside the dream that you have to attend to, like answering the door or telephone when you're napping.

Australian Aborigine shamans spent a great deal of time in an altered state which they referred to as Dreamtime. Being in Dreamtime was a tool that allowed the wise men and women to predict events, travel in the astral plane, and perform certain healing rituals. Dreamtime was considered a creative state where the normal rules of time and space did not exist. The concept of Dreamtime corresponds with the Void in Aborigine creation legends as the source of life. This seems to be pretty strong evidence that you don't have to be asleep to make use of your dream states.

A waking vision is not the same as a dream. It is more like a hallucination, a dream with the power to intrude on the perceptual screen of the social self when wide awake. This is not entertainment like a drug reaction; it's more like a nightmare in intensity but can be positive and even fun. This can be brought on empathically when sharing something exciting with awakened companions. I've had that happen with Veronica Moran while partying, and Kevin Millis while swimming. Veronique (nickname) and I were standing in a hallway when suddenly a tunnel formed between us and we both stepped inside and were no longer at the party. Kevin and I were snorkeling in southern California when we both started to have what Maslow would call a peak experience. We were both seeing on the same spectrum and could describe to each other what we were experiencing.

I've talked with married couples who sometimes share each other's minds. It's not that uncommon. The Russians supposedly have done a lot of research in this area. Now that the Iron Curtain has collapsed, we may get to examine what they've done with telemetry, telepathy, clairvoyance, and so forth. I used to be pretty skeptical of this whole area of investigation. Now I'm skeptically curious.

Waking visions also seem to be part of the meditative experience, as I described in the chapters concerning the kundalini. There may also be a link with past-life experience, spirits, and/or genetic memory, which I tend to discount even given my personal experiences (I prefer not to wade in those waters, though I seem to get splashed from time to time). Dr. Rich Grant once found himself immersed in a cavalry charge in France of a few centuries back. Suzanne Carlson dreamed of herself as her father as a young man in World War II London during the bombings. I've been on a high platform watching troops in strange uniforms pass in review (this was not a pleasant vision), as well as been a trader with bronze spearheads poling a log canoe with a leather sail. The feeling is you are wide awake, but what you are watching is a dream that is, was, or can be part of you.

Dreamwork can also be a spontaneous response to receiving higher energy from a master of chi kung or someone who has gone through the kundalini and figured out what to do with themselves besides head for a rubber room. I'm thinking of the example of Arlene Hill, a theatre student. Blake Poindexter (hoshin sandan) and I wired her up with meridian massage at a party when she was dating Mark Robinson, one of our blue belts. We both dumped a lot of energy into her as we were working out her kinks.

Arlene codified a phenomenon that I hadn't really thought much about. She was completely on her own, as she and Mark broke up soon after and she wasn't training with us, so she had no idea what to expect or what we had done to her. One thing she definitely didn't expect was the vivid increase in the intensity of her dreams as her body began the process of rewiring to handle the higher energy we had dumped in her. She personally blamed me and particularly resented being chased from her loft in a dream by a shape-changer which caused her to fall and break her foot. As Arlene's energy escalated she was also presented with the problem of how to deal with her suddenly much greater attraction to men as well as a quantum jump in her performance skills. She was also confused by the admiring approach of satanists, as well as meditators and yogis who had never shown any interest in her before. Her broken foot kept her from blowing off the excess energy through dance, and she was not interested in the men she was drawing to her flame, so her elevation was not without some internal pain from overloaded biocircuitry. There is something to the power of virgins.

When I was working for General Motors and living on a little lake, my neighbor across the way was a nurse. I asked her if she meditated or knew therapeutic touch. She didn't and wanted to learn. One week while her husband was attending a conference so she didn't have to devote her evenings to him, I taught her how to meditate and give meridian massage as well as read auras and use therapeutic touch. (This can only be done by energy exchange.) About a week later, she told me she had the following dream. Her husband and she were at a restaurant when a group of Japanese dressed as businessmen struck him down and kidnapped her. They hid her away in a large stone castle and she was feeling very lost and helpless. She was taken to a room to be interrogated by a large group of men. While they were distracted by torturing her, I walked into the room. I changed into a large black bird with claws for hands and feet and long sharp bill. I tore into the back of the group and began shredding them with great glee. I killed them all. I then returned her to her husband. At the time of this dream she had no knowledge of ninjutsu and certainly wasn't aware of an esoteric piece of information like tengu are ninja are birds. Her healing skills improved and her doctor wanted to take her with him when he moved into private practice.

Steven, a student of Mark's, once had a dream about me after we had worked out together at Mark's place on Bear Lake. Blake and I were demonstrating how hard you could hit with chi, and Steven may have been cannon fodder once or twice in the course of the demo. It's interesting having third-generation students as you don't have any idea what they know, or don't know, not being their teacher. Steven told Mark he'd had the following dream.

"I was sitting in a large banquet hall. There were many people there and we were waiting for the speaker. Finally, the huge doors at the end of the hall opened and in walked Dr. Morris. He was escorted by four beautiful women, each of a different race. They were very solicitous of his comfort. His talk was about the importance of conserving your sexual energy which was very funny since the women did not seem to be very helpful in that direction." As Steve is a very handsome young man, he thought he would attempt a pick-up of Old Baldy's escort. "When I approached the women, they poked fun at me and slandered my manhood. It was very embarrassing. They said that at my level of potency they would be jailed for manslaughter if we got it on." Steve knew nothing about the Yellow Emperor and his Court of Lovelies and neither did Mark at that time. I had not yet given him the *Big Red Book* (Douglas and Slinger's *Sexual Secrets*).

When Kevin and I were giving Earth and Fire seminars on his turf south of L.A., a higher-ranking American ninja decided he could attend for free, take over to give a couple of advanced lessons, and probably rip off a few of our students as rank hath its privilege. He showed up late in the afternoon of the second day after I'd spent the first day teaching the participants how to see and feel energy. He had only met me once before at a Tai Kai and had no idea what my skills and interests were. (It must be remembered that in Togakure Ryu Ninjutsu some of the masters are much more physically talented than mentally. Some have never shown any interest in the soft side of the art; some who are thick as bricks refute their own experience and say it doesn't exist; and there are a few whose level of enlightenment allows them to attempt to fake it. *Genjutsu,* or faking skills for professional reasons, is not denigrated by the system but can be a necessary survival skill for duping the naive.)

Anyway, this boob starts telling the students to watch how his energy moves up the chakras as he performs some techniques. I had to warn the class to remember Hatsumi's dictum concerning trusting your own senses and primary sources. When the day was finished I summarized the learnings and invited those who weren't exhausted after two twelve-hour days to come party with Kevin and me in Malibu. The visiting master got to sleep alone in his truck in the parking lot. He told Kevin he had terrible nightmares and could hardly sleep at all that night. I have noticed over the years that his taijutsu has improved enormously, but since he is not a friend I'm not aware of the state of his ego. I've not spoken to him in years.

You can usually tell when a dream is not yours, as the symbols and feelings will be wildly different from your own. Now, intruding into someone else's dream requires that you know how to get on that person's or group's wavelength, or you have shared energy and are "in" that person so you can go visit your energy baby. Rather like some of the experiences that twins report. Most people regard the penetration of their dream in about the same way a victim regards rape. It is scary to realize that someone else can share your dream. This is very different from dreaming about someone. This is being visited by an alien presence in your most inner and sacred being.

It is probably a good idea to approach dreamwork with caution. It's an intense form of telepathy. When I returned from England after taking Suzanne Carlson through the kundalini, she would show up in dreams and dreamtime. That was very pleasant since I like Suzanne. I talked with her old boyfriend and he said that she'd been able to do that with him for a long time. It's a different matter when the appearance is unexpected. He wrote a song for his Chicago rock band, The Mean Reds, that is quite popular in the dance bars, called "Get Out of My Mind!" It's about how difficult it is to shake the witch-lover's spell. A lot of people seem to empathize with his anger.

There is a ninja story concerning a high-level physical practitioner who wanted to learn how to use dreams. His teacher trusted him to use the information for self- protection; instead he decided to intimidate the samurai he worked for by sending him nightmares. He dropped hints so that the samurai would realize the source of his night terrors and bribe him appropriately to win back his peace of mind. The samurai chose another route of continuously assigning his ninja subordinate to increasingly dangerous jobs until he was severely injured in an explosion that could have been ignorance or sabotage. Only the ninja's superb taijutsu prevented him from being killed and disfigured. The samurai then truly feared and retained him, as he survived where lesser men would have died. When I told my master boxer friend John Yono this story, he said, "I would have sent the nightmare and then rescued the samurai from what I sent, building his gratitude." John's is a more Christian viewpoint.

Before the Texas Tai Kai in 1991, Hatsumi-san came to me in a dream. It was in the early morning hours when I like to meditate while lying in bed. Often the male sexual energy is higher in the morning, and this is a good time to draw it off your testicles if your spouse is tired. I was lying beside my wife in that state between dream and waking when Hatsumi and a beautiful Japanese woman appeared in the buff before my surprised eyes. It had been over a year since I'd seen him and I'm pretty certain he was in Japan. He began to speak to me in telepathic English baby talk.

"You can love me even more by loving her," he said as he gestured broadly and dumped his energy into his female companion. It did not require a degree in cross-cultural nonverbal communication to notice her enthusiasm. Esotericists might find this visit a manifestation of sadhana complete with dakini or khadroma. (Look it up.) Anyway, it scared the hell out of me. I retaliated by sending a dream date for his turkey, owl, and dogs.

Often a spirit will approach you during dream states. They seem to be strongest around midnight. A guiding spirit may be considered an angel if you're a Christian or an ally if you're into American Indian spirit lore. I personally don't think it is a good idea to attack them like Jacob in the Bible story. They cannot cross the dimensional plane unless you feed them energy, and you can't do that unless you know how to transfer chi or are so scared you kick into fear and terror mode, which radiates all over the place and the boogie gets it for free. It's more interesting to make it a friend or pet. Kick back, relax, match breaths, and observe carefully.

Pay close attention to the feelings, as this is in no way an intellectual exercise. If the spirit gets uppity—eat it. Just inhale it with your tongue and recycle it through your orbits. It can be quite a rush. (See the yogic asana or pose called the lion. You might remember the tongue as an organ of spiritual transfer from your tantric practice.) The stronger spirit wins. All the crap about how powerful they are is propaganda to frighten the foolish and superstitious. This is a creature of energy and breath. It's lighter than air. Its only hope of survival is in not being noticed when on our plane. It's curious as to how you got over into its realm while you are obviously still in the material world. It remembers being carnate. It's happy to share information, particularly if you're willing to share energy. No human sacrifices necessary if you've developed your own inexhaustible source of living energy through chi kung.

You probably know as much about dreamwork as I do. It's a new interest for me. Toff, Blake, and the Hoosier element of hoshin fancy their dream skills. The basics relate to lucid dreaming. Higher energy is necessary for sending over distances. The periods just before waking or going to sleep allow access to nonordinary lower brain functions similar to meditation. Visual exchange does seem to work better at night. Sending down works better than sending up. Interchange between compatibles or equals is quite vivid. Indian shamans would often use animals to transport their spirit in dreamwork.

Recently after a workout I went to a massage therapist I've been teaching the hoshin meditation skills to see if she could release some of the tighter fascia in my legs and hips as I've never been satisfied with my flexibility. She said there was some surprising tightness and worked my legs through all kinds of funny little lifts and stretches to break things a little looser. It felt great. I told her the story about being on Ilana Rubenfeld's table and the oatmeal abuse. She thought it was funny and remarked how women often do damage unawares. Psychoanalysis often reveals the beginning of female-hating as a response to careless mothering, as if adolescent rejections weren't enough. We talked about Bly's men's groups and I expressed my opinion that he will probably do for fathering what Freud did for mothering in the long run. He's a better poet than shaman/psychologist.

That night in my dreams I was weeping and recognizing how much I missed the only woman with whom I have ever been romantically in love. She was twenty-some years younger than I and had her own life to create. I tried very hard to keep from connecting her to me and when it finally happened was so astounded by the depth of connection and experience granted to enlightened lovers that I lost all semblance or need for distance and just launched myself at her. I have had considerable erotic experience of the fairer sex over the years, even taking the vows of matrimony twice, but had never come across telepathic love-making, sharing energy, and being what she described in her inexperience as "compatible and passionate."

It has been years since I've seen her, though little things happen daily that cause me to think of her. We did not part well or happily. I showed her my very worst and succeeded in driving her away. It was painful and stupid on my part, but the age difference seemed as monumental to me then from a teacher's perspective as race to a bigot or IQ to an intellectual. It does not seem strange to me that she would be released by the stretching of the hips and pelvis. Dreams are one of the doorways to the body's knowledge. Sometimes the dream provides the only acceptable release.

Nowadays there are all sorts of "revolutionary tools for higher consciousness." I have tried most of these toys over the years and have come to the firm conclusion that higher consciousness comes from your genitals and brainstem, not your cortex, and you will be much happier with the results of meditation on the microcosmic orbit and breathwork. You have to develop the initial power before you can reach out and touch something with any degree of consistency. At this writing I've come into very interesting and real contact with Shiva, Tara and/or Sophia (who would seem to be interchangeable with Ningobble of the Many Eyes), Jesus, Kali, Kobo Daishi, Athena, and the Yellow Emperor, to mention those consciousnesses that have recognizable characteristics, and some others that were beyond me to recognize and a few that I ate. As I find religion ridiculous for the most part and was not drunk, stoned, or on acid at the time, I suggest an attitude of friendly observation and willingness to share as the proper approach to spirit contact, as opposed to worship and fawning.

All hallucinations are supposed to be part of you or a product of your own mind. Share and tell. It might just be your left lobe after all. In dreamtime anything is possible, and there seem to be some interesting problems with time if not space and distance. Some master-level practitioners of Shaolin Kempo or Sillum Kung Fu are rumored to be able to cross time barriers through meditation and breath control. Nobody in my circle of friends has figured that one out. The immortals live on in dreamtime.

See you in your dreams.

Chapter Fifteen

Magic, Crystals, Talismans, and Swords

THE FOCUS OF intention is the basis of all magic. There is "one thing that allows you to learn the 10,000 things" continually referred to but seldom explained in Eastern esoteric literature; that is meditation. The type of meditation required to truly focus intent, however, is a step beyond focusing on a mantra or going into relaxation response. It is going into your self to awaken your true Self, which connects to the Universal. Internal practice is necessary to affecting the external reality.

The Chinese practitioners of chi kung, the swamis of India, the Zen roshi, and the ninja are prominent examples of those who pursue enlightenment or awakening. Awakening is simply waking up your id, shadow, or true self. Enlightenment is the biological process of rejuvenating your hormone system. The side effects of obtaining enlightenment are called in Sanskrit "siddhi." In the context of Buddhist yoga or *Vajrayana* (perfect mastery over the body and forces of nature) there are eight ordinary siddhis: 1. the sword that renders unconquerable; 2. the elixir for the eyes that makes gods visible; 3. fleetness in running; 4. invisibility; 5. the life essence that preserves youth; 6. the ability to fly, levitate, and/or project onto the astral plane; 7. the ability to make certain medicines; 8. power over the world of spirits and demons.

The order appears to be hierarchical. Some of these can also be described as mind-reading, clairvoyance, empathy, materialization, levitation, making things invisible, and entering other bodies. I have yet to witness what I consider true materialization or levitation; astral projection is trippy enough for me.

Many wise men and women say that no one can attain enlightenment without the assistance of a perfect master. It strikes me as difficult but not impossible to a good researcher willing to take some chances. This isn't the tenth century. This is America. The libraries are open, if not filled. My own experience has led me to believe the preserved descriptions concerning these powers are somewhat rhetorically exaggerated, and human beings should not be overly concerned with fantasies like perfection. Murphy seems to share my opinion.

All these powers seem supernatural if you haven't learned how to do them or opened yourself up to the experience. All science appears as magic to the ignorant. All the great sages agree that they are also just distractions to obtaining enlightenment or absolute truth, as attachment to a particular siddhi is an obstacle in the way of spiritual development. What that means is, if you waste all your time trying to learn how to read other people's minds or master the secret sword techniques instead of working on your own damn self, you have missed the point of the exercise— rather like a psychologist who breaks off his or her own analysis. However, it is easy to speculate uses of such powers for a sage or gatherer of intelligence.

Another problem concerning the pursuit of enlightenment is the identification of a legitimate teacher, as well as separation from the teacher once the goal has been attained or particular lesson learned. Perhaps in these days it is more accurate to say avoiding attachment to the teacher as you attempt to solve your own inner puzzle. Most traditional teachers expect devotion. It's where the word "devotee" comes from, meaning disciple or deshi. It's not an American concept nor is devotion necessary to the biological process of enlightenment, but it can make life easier for the teacher and the student if the relationship is understood from the start.

Enlightenment is differentiated from the eight ordinary siddhi as the sole extraordinary or supreme siddhi. It's number nine. And its expression is as diverse as the many-petaled lotus used to represent its accomplishment in India. The enlightened individual is supposed to be able to demonstrate mastery of the common eight from his or her locus of control, rendering a new and positive form to the dark and ancient magic. The meditative techniques I've described are virtually the same in Taoism, Kriya yoga, Kokoro, Kabbalah, Esoteric Christianity, and Sufism. Manifestation may differ according to the practice, but the true practice has to do with going within and working on yourself and your breath following the light—not drawing pentagrams on the floor that represent internal states and standing in them while bellowing in languages you don't understand.

Kuji (mudra) and *Juji* (spirituality) and similar practices are well documented in esoteric literature. A helpful book, *Where the Spirits Ride The Wind: Trance Journeys and other Ecstatic Experiences* by Felicitas D. Goodman (Indiana University, 1990), lays out some 30 postures that are especially trance-inducing. Some are very similar to the moving kamae of ninjutsu; others are much more American Indian. Kuji can be used to shift the flow of chi energy from the normal patterns through the meridians, and one who is pursuing enlightenment should explore those avenues. They definitely affect the brain, particularly the cerebellum. Hayes's workshops on the kuji are very well received. Once internal energy is transformed, it can be externalized and that is real magic. However, things aren't always what they seem, and the ancient gods felt and feel it a duty to twist the wish of a power seeker. What you see may just be what you get. Transformation is a two-lane highway.

Crystals have a long history of medical and esoteric use. It has been my experience that plain old quartz crystal in its various colors along with aquamarines, tourmalines, and moonstones may be the only stones worth wearing on the body. The harder the stone the less charge it can carry and the lesser its ability to affect a gland. Quartz can hold a charge if you run your chi into it. It also has a subtle electrical field around it, so that if you wear one over your thyroid it stimulates the gland. The kings and queens of yore wore crystals not gems in their crowns to stimulate the occult powers. Thrones usually had a giant stone hidden in the seat to stimulate the genitals. (The throne of England had a huge red carbuncle that is now kept in the Tower of London.) Gems came along when money started to get confused with power.

Lovers in the Renaissance gave each other crystal rings to wear on the water meridian (kidney, ancient seat of the emotions) or third finger of the left hand after they had charged them with their feelings for the other person. A nice way to reinforce affection. The ring wearer would tend to think of the giver more often. You can see how easily sentiment can be perverted by price.

Wearing a crystal helps to harmonize your energy fields, but the clarity, size, or color are of little consequence. Where you hang it is more important, as you want proximity to the governing meridians or organs you wish to stimulate. A cheapie held on by a piece of leather can do the job as well as the "occultly perfect stone" in a jeweler's setting. What is important is whether you feel energy in the stone. Many people will disagree with my experience, but we follow our own placebos.

Once the target gland is functioning properly, you will probably find wearing the crystal no longer has any effect. Reactivated hormonal or endocrine glands seem to want to keep working if given a little gentle encouragement from breath and crystal. The body enjoys being healthy. Subtle energy techniques like this can take a little more time but also seem to outlast a kick start. Clear the crystal when you no longer need it and give it to a friend.

Once you have developed chi you can easily pass some of your charge into wood. The favorite *hanbo* (walking stick) becomes charged with the intention of the handler. I've noticed considerable difference in the feel of *bokken* (hardwood practice swords) and hanbo of students and teachers when I chanced to pick them up. It's a fun exercise in sensitivity. Can you tell whose stick is whose? (It is also considered extremely rude to handle or step over another's weapons or practice weapons without permission. You should adopt a look of innocent wonder as you drain or sabotage a piece with your foot.)

This same principle of chi transference applies to the making of works of art and religious objects. The artist channels his or her feelings into the work. If the artist's intent is strong you can actually feel the energy he or she put into manufacturing the work (ritual magic is part of the sword-making art in Japan). This principle even applies to letters and handwritten documents. Supposedly information is passed by the touch of the scroll when it is made by a powerful mage who pours his intent into the medium as well as the message. Hatsumi-soke hand-creates all promotion diplomas for Bujinkan. I like to pass my hand over mine from time to time just to get a feel of the man.

When I was in England visiting Suzanne Carlson we went to the Victoria and Albert Museum to check out the Japanese swords encased there. Two of the swords could push our hands back from the glass when we followed the energy flow. We both thought that was pretty special, so we looked to see who made them and when. Both of the pushy swords were older than the others and made by priests. They were all magnificent examples of the sword-maker's art. Doing detail work can fix the mind but it is the emotion that creates the art. This may account for the tales of lucky, life-giving swords and unlucky swords whose owners seemed to come to a nasty end. The sword test in ninjutsu when performed with a live sword is supposed to be done always with a virgin sword so that complete neutrality of outcome is observed. I once heard Hatsumi say, "Buddha men would only use their swords for right things!"

There is a broken sword displayed in shihan Tetsuji Ishizuka's dojo in Kashiwa. Hatsumi broke it with his bare hands. They took it to be assayed and the analysis said the steel around the break had strangely crystallized. We all know about the hardness and strangeness of some Japanese swords. I have an old sword made by Yoshida Tamekichi of Seki. It's a night sword, which means the blade is mottled and smoky in appearance so that it's hard to see. Same principle as bluing a knife or gun. I bought it from an antique dealer for $75 as it was pretty beat up and the bloodstains in the officer handle wrappings weren't particularly attractive. Its owner probably didn't make it home. Every time I tried to sharpen it or clean it up, I'd get cut—once to the bone on my left thumb knuckle. I read a biography of Tesshu (one of the last great samurai swordsmen to achieve enlightenment) and decided to try running energy into the blade as well as meditating with it in my lap. One night as I was meditating the sword became very cold and a woman's voice spoke to me saying, "You keep that ninja *to* (short straight-bladed sword favored by boat warriors) beside your bed instead of me. How can you be such a fool? Don't you know I deserve better treatment than this?!"

I got up, moved the *to* out of the bedroom, and put her beside my bed. She has been light and easy to handle ever since. I haven't been cut since. I had her scabbard and handle decorated by my mystical jeweler friend for a whopping fee. I had her nose redone even though it dropped her value as a bushido collector's item by ten thousand dollars. The sword sometimes seems to move about me on her own when I do sword drills as a form of compassionate compensation. I don't have the faintest idea how a swordmaker trapped a female spirit in a sword three hundred years ago. Given some of the cutting drills used by the samurai to test swords, such as hacking up prisoners, I don't think I want to know. I'm just happy to own such an interesting artifact. I call her Lydia, after Kenneth Robert's wonderful book *Lydia Bailey.* My cynical Crowley-following friend says she's probably some old whore who tried to short-sheet a samurai.

The swords and hanbo are but two examples. Chi can be passed on to other objects if you want to work real hard, I suppose. Healers will often charge water for their clients to drink. The clients sometime report it makes them feel as if they had drunk a little wine. Who knows what charging up your Macintosh might accomplish if you're a writer. But it's probably more beneficial to work on your typing skills than the creation of esoteric bugs. The telephone is more reliable than the telepath. It is probably not wise to encourage the ghosts in machines.

Chapter Sixteen

Spirits . . . Things that go bump in the night

There are a number of books concerning enlightenment that treat the experience as religious, and that's fair since most of the literature in the West comes from Buddhist translations or pseudoscientific investigations by occultists. (It might be recalled that the founder of Zen, Da Mo, the Bodhidharma, is the same fellow credited with beginning Shaolin Kung Fu and developing marrow-washing and brain-energizing chi kung.) For a Christian perspective on enlightenment and meditative practice I strongly recommend Meister Eckhart or St. John of the Cross. Even more interesting might be the *Gospel of St. Thomas,* recently dug up at Nag Hammadi; it's the only gospel written by an actual witness, as the other Gospels were rewritten long after Christ's death and based on hearsay. My understanding is that it was considered apocrypha and did not survive beyond the fifth century as a source of doctrine.

There also is a burgeoning body of literature concerning shamanism that is gaining in popularity; much of it flows out of the somewhat questionable work of Carlos Castaneda (who went a bit native) and more scientific investigators such as Doore and Harner. Back at the turn of the century we had the Golden Dawn crowd, Gurdjieff, and wild fellows like Crowley. Some left rather interesting cookbooks. My own experiences following no particular teacher but being perfectly happy to experiment on myself have left me convinced that no single practice has a corner on the market. If you want to do it yourself, chi kung is a valid, scientifically replicable system for achieving not just incredible strength and health but much of what the Hindu refer to as siddhi, Westerners as magic, occultists as power, and Taoists as the Way, or in the general vernacular—enlightenment.

All of these folks, myself included, regard or regarded themselves as sane, responsible presenters of useful information. I'm sharing my experience. Nobody taught me. All shortcomings are my own. If you don't like what I'm putting in the public record, then get to work on your own. You don't know until you've experienced. When I have a problem I go to an expert. If I can't speak his language, I observe and try to find competent translators. There seems to be a lot better stuff around these days than when Madame Blavatsky or William James were writing. My belief system was more shaped by Poul Anderson, Andrea Norton, and Robert Heinlein than any of the above.

When I was a graduate student at Penn State, I had a conversation with Norris Durham, a physical anthropologist, about a paper by someone positing the hypothesis that dominant males in protohuman primate groups achieved their status by being able to shock their subordinates—something akin to electric eels. We laughed ourselves silly over that one. I'd yet to be exposed to the internal arts, and chi was still a foreign concept.

Modern man is a lot larger than our Medieval forebears, yet the knights were able to dress up in heavy (by our standards) armor and go after each other with clubs and swords for days on end. That kind of endurance strikes me as chi-driven and leads me to the conclusion that the Chinese royal families and Shaolin monks weren't alone in their discoveries. Orientals only had to contend with ignorance, not the Inquisition, book burning, the Dark Ages, fundamentalists, Luddites, and Puritan Roundheads— challenges that eradicated most Western esoteric knowledge. What was saved was in code to protect the human alchemists, and before long the codes were followed, not the hidden meaning. However, we did get chemistry and astronomy.

Western materialism is pretty hard to compete with, as it is a lot more fun and delivers faster feedback than working on taking conscious control of your body's electrical system (or mastering the secrets of Holy Water). I've found all the techniques in chi kung described in European alchemical texts, and the symbols for transformation are almost universal. All you need to know is in the Grail quests. What was that Green Knight all about? Islam has Khezr and Sufis.

We've all heard of the strength of the insane, of manic or maniacal strength. There is a great little horror movie called *Eyes of Fire* about an Irish faerie in North America around 1750. The story is told from the viewpoint of the observing children and occasionally shifts to what the mad girl or faerie sees. I found the movie quite remarkable because I have seen through her eyes. Whoever was responsible for that script did excellent research. Everyone who has ever watched it was mesmerized by the story. Thomas Szazz, the famous psychologist, has written that much of what passes as insanity is only extremes of behavior and interpretation. Anyway, when the hormonal systems supercharge for fight or flight, the brain gets a load of chemicals that can wildly alter your perception of the world as you knew it. If you are fearful, your focus is narrowed to all that can go wrong and you plunge into paranoia. Your imagination fills in the gaps of your perception and you hallucinate all that frightens you. If you cannot discriminate between the real and the imagined, you may act on your "feelings." You have discovered Hell and no one else seems to share it.

If your viewpoint is positive and you are loving, the perceptual world that emerges is much different. Dr. Abraham Maslow described it as "peak experience" and practically everyone has one from time to time. Your world is beautiful and so are all your acquaintances. You move with grace and power, as there are no fears or barriers to your accomplishment. Your hallucinations may take on a Walt Disney flavor. If you start having too much fun and see yourself as God, even though your vision is benevolent and harmless, you too can be given the rubber room. Yin and yang. Moderation in all things seems to be the Way. (I recommend attempting associative preference for a demigod at first.) As you gain control of your hormonal system through proper exercise of the breath and posture, the changes will affect your total persona, and until you learn to relax into it, delusions of grandeur is the price you pay for lack of humility. You get it (the Self) under control or it gets you. You're still you, just more amplified, with some additional talents and viewpoints that very few people you know share unless you're an adept or an esoteric martial artist of high level. You are playing in the fields of dreams and the stuff of legends.

As one of the early changes, you become more nocturnal and see farther into the infrared spectrum, allowing you not only to see the heat envelope around others but also where their energy fields are strongest. This is a considerable advantage when applying shiatsu or using therapeutic touch. After you have learned to "see" energy as a side effect of controlling binocular vision and enhancing your hormonal or chakra system through relaxed breathing techniques, the energy around people's bodies will be readily apparent even in bright light as long as the background is relatively flat. Fortunately most people don't have much energy or the faintest idea how to use it, so you're probably further ahead to keep your extra bit of info to yourself, as most others don't see it. This is well described in the healing literature concerning alternative medicine.

I recall once being described by a ninja acquaintance as "someone who sees what others can't." No, that's too nice. What she actually said was, "Oh, you're him, you're Dr. Morris. I've heard of you. You can see things that other people don't and there are rumors you're into green belt sacrifices. No thank you, I'll find another training partner." Such is life in the big city and the relatively small world of martial artists.

People who have strong energy project their id into their aura and it can be seen. If you can't see it, you can certainly feel it. Hayes describes a time when Tanemura dropped him with an energy strike, and I've "seen" Hatsumi use energy a number of times. At the shidoshi training, celebrating his thirtieth anniversary as grandmaster, he threw a rather arrogant young Israeli godan, and asked him to explain what had just happened to him. The Israeli's comment after the throw was, "I tried to hit Hatsumi, everything went black, then I was in the air and landed on my head. I don't know how I got from the punch to the *tatami*" (special mats built into the floors of a dojo). He was quite perplexed.

What I saw was Hatsumi take the energy from his punch, add it to his own, and send it back into the young man, overloading his circuits/channels/meridians and causing him to momentarily black out while Hatsumi completed the throw with his usual aplomb and amazing grace. Hatsumi then rebalanced the fallen warrior as he helped him to his feet. I have seen Leo Sebregst, a Wu Shu SiGung, perform in a similar fashion. The ability to use sexual energy for both attack and healing is quite rare in the West but a common legendary theme in the East, where the link between medicine and martial arts is tradition. Both Hatsumi and Nagato are bone doctors. (Sebregst only uses the healing side under duress; he is not a medical practitioner.) Some of the stories concerning Hatsumi's cures and healings border on the miraculous if one does not comprehend energy use. The stories are verifiable.

Yoki no kamae, kyojutsu, or *Yojutsu* (the ability to project "weird airs" or illusions) is one of the side effects of having developed your chi. In chapter thirteen, "Mirror, mirror . . .," I describe the passive use of this skill. Yojutsu requires the projection or channeling of intention. A skilled adept can project energy and faces to frighten an attacker, or encircle him with unexpected weirdness or bolts of energy and feelings. Hindu adepts describe this as directing *chitta* (life force), and its use is a closely guarded secret of yogic magicians. However, Ormond McGill in his book *Hypnotism and Mysticism of India* (Westwood, 1979) provides useful descriptions and techniques. Interestingly enough, this type of phenomena can best be discerned in dim light or darkness. Bright sunlight or electric lighting can wash out the projection, but light does not wash out the effect. The Tibetans refer to this as "creating *tulpus*," and supposedly a master can create an illusion so real that you can engage it in conversation. I've never seen that, but I read a research paper paid for by the C.I.A. back in the seventies that discussed the possibilities. What I have seen is similar but not so grandiose, and on one level resembles channeling and on another is probably a side effect of energy transfer.

A powerful person's aura has a bright corona that extends out from the head and shoulders approximately six inches to a foot. If they usually think in a particular pattern this will be revealed by color shades in the field. A normal person's corona is approximately a quarter-inch to an inch thick and diffuses quickly as it extends from the body. A person who has been working with their energy or spiritual development does not diffuse so quickly but is surrounded by a fairly coherent field that extends outward from three to thirty feet. It looks like a cloud of mist. It usually appears as a halo or glow about the individual. Usually the close-to-the-body corona is all you'll see without practice or optimal conditions. It will occasionally be picked up by television cameras if the angles are right.

Esotericists have names for these fields, such as the "soul body" and so forth. They believe this field is what survives after death and in reality is your true self and the basis of most religions. Healers perceive it as living energy and use it to stimulate the damaged cells of their clients to return to healthy growth. It is a gift of the spirit that heals. A teacher exchanges energy with his or her student, transferring the feeling of a particular action. What is transferred depends on the skill of the teacher and the receptive skills of the student. Teachers in the esoteric martial arts are revered by their students, because the student recognizes that without the gift of energy or spirit they would never have been able to develop on their own. At some point the teacher has to cut the students loose so they can develop their own talents free from dependency. Those that are self-taught often think they have succeeded from lack of peer feedback and must guard against paranoia with humility.

I attended a *Pak Kua* (internal organ strengthening techniques) seminar taught by one of Mantak Chia's students in the Detroit suburbs and was quite impressed by the fields emanating from his body. I almost cracked up at a number of points when he would demonstrate a technique for us and say, "Mantak Chia stands behind this," and a ghostly apparition of Mantak Chia would appear in his aura standing behind him. After the seminar was over I gave him a quick lesson in aura viewing in exchange for some of the useful insights he'd given me. Giri.

Sellers Smith, a student of ninjutsu and a martial arts friend, attended a Common Boundary convention in Washington, D.C., with me where a renowned healer was presenting. She is a channel who uses therapeutic touch, energy transformation of the chakras, and sound vibration for psychic healing. While she was working on a volunteer from the audience she allowed her guiding entity to come through her. Sellers and I both saw her aura expand to include this big ball of energy that wasn't there before. It appeared as energy, not as a recognizable person. At least not to us. When my student Dr. Richard Grant studied with Leo Sebregst in South Africa, I was surprised to find Leo's head looking out at me from Rick's aura one evening when we were cracking jokes in Johannesburg. Seems he likes a good laugh, too.

Kevin Millis was showing me some *naginata* techniques (sword blade on a *bo* staff, usually used by women or shamans) one night in his Irvine dojo. His skills and control were so overwhelming that if I weren't a hobbyist (thus having no pride) I would never have dared to pick up a spear again. He was giving me the worst thrashing of my life without hurting me or even causing much pain, but everything I tried to do was absorbed, put me off balance, and resulted in me being crushed to the floor with some extremely vulnerable part of my anatomy exposed to his blade. It was an impeccable demonstration of weapon mastery. As I was having my butt so thoroughly kicked I still can't properly describe it, I was filled with this feeling of complete and utter terror for the error of my ways for even thinking to strike at a teacher. (He was pissing me off.) As these waves of remorse washed over me I shifted my vision and "saw" a Japanese Noh dancer complete with mask, long white hair, splendid costume, and whirling naginata moving with some of the wildest taijutsu I've ever seen. Every time this entity moved through Kevin to do something totally beyond my ability to predict or respond, it would rear back in a victory dance, imitating a rock and roll guitarist doing a heavy metal riff (Kevin was once a rock and roll guitarist and still plays professionally) rather like MTV from hell. Then it would come after me again, flipping me out by wielding a long, giant stone penis and attempting to crush me with it. The first three of the five hellish crimes in Buddhism are matricide, patricide, and the murder of an enlightened teacher. I was giving him my best shot. He didn't seem to be holding anything back. I have seldom been more frightened and yet had more fun. If you think you're a good martial artist, this kind of a lesson is horrorshow dark horse indeed!

Hatsumi says the spirits of the tradition flow through the grandmaster, and this little vignette concerning Kevin's boogie man might illustrate what that means. I later asked Kevin if he knew what a Noh dancer was or had ever attended classical Noh theater. He said he didn't have any idea what I was talking about. Seeing the spirit do air guitar maneuvers with the naginata convinced me it was having a good time, even if I wasn't. The exchange between Kevin and the Noh dancer was impressive. (Some Noh dancers were considered to be shamans. Actors and dancers were two of the traditional disguises of the ninja involved in intelligence gathering.)

This is yojutsu or mental projection as performed with a spirit guide and probably a little gift from Hatsumi or just the luck of the Taoist draw while wandering around in Japan. According to the ancient Taoists, spirits are attracted by the enlightened and align themselves appropriately—a spiritual illustration of "The Law of Attraction." Healers get healers, scholars get scholars, and warriors get warriors. The more powerful you are, the more spirits you attract. My hypothesis is that the guiding spirit achieved enlightenment in its life and now gets to play, but I've no idea as to how to test it other than check out of this existence, and I'm having too much fun for that. I do know that yojutsu is real and most people who have chi can project feelings and faces before them that can be seen in the dark. Probably explains the boogie men reported by children.

When Hillsdale College informed me my job was being eliminated, my second wife informed she wanted a divorce, as she knew there was no way I could stay in Jonesville and make a decent living. She wanted to stay there because the kids were happy in their schools. I was filled with this incredible grief because I'd truly loved this particular job and felt I had learned how to be a very good father and loving husband. I thought my family would go with me. I was used to moving and starting over. Preachers' kids move every five years. At that time my student Suzanne Carlson told me she could feel my sorrow palpably across a distance of more than fifty feet. She said it was hard to do anything when I was feeling so sad. Bad vibes, passive yojutsu.

When I was traveling with Hayes on one of his ninja tours of old Japan we visited many interesting sites and temples important to the historical ninja. One of the experiences that had a powerful effect on me was a visit to a particular temple in which the energy was the color and feeling appropriate to what the temple was dedicated to. Supposedly this is a skill of the Shinto priests in site energy selection. It is an art and service for charge among certain Chinese sects and Shinto priests that previous to this jaunt I'd thought of as charlatans. Temples for strength had red energy; one for water/female was orange. Togakushi was green and blue and white. It certainly surprised me. I've been in a lot of old buildings in Europe and Africa and never picked up a thing. Of course at that time in my life I wasn't capable of looking, so maybe I shouldn't be that impressed, but I've checked out a few American institutions since and was disappointed with the exception of the Lincoln Memorial. The only other source of wild energy like that which I've experienced was at Joshua Tree National Monument, climbing with Kevin Millis, or where there is a lot of quartz crystal in the ground.

One of the interesting places we visited in Japan was Koyasan, home of Kobo Daishi, founder of Shingon Buddhism. There was a celebration of his spirit's annual return to earth one night when we were there. It seems to me it corresponds to our All Hallows Eve. Together with Michael Fenster, a very smart young medical student who is now a shodan in ninjutsu and a sandan in hoshin, I wanted to observe this event. We decided to walk through an amazing old graveyard and memorial ground that is a huge park in the center of the city. There are memorials to the forty-seven *ronin*, to Musashi, and to American dead from a plane shot down in WWII, as well as aborted children, poets, shogun, and samurai, all interred together or at least recognized as a part of the history of this mountain city. Graves and memorials piled on top of each other, from ancient to modern, sitting cheek to jowl, rooted in the rocks and giant trees for a thousand years.

A young Zen monk, Kuboda, was staying with the Mikkyos so that he could give us a lecture in English and a demonstration of how his Renzai sect taught meditation. He told us we were nuts to go through that graveyard at night without protection. Not being superstitious, we ignored his heartfelt warnings, not having the faintest idea what protection might be necessary as we were skilled martial artists and could probably handle anyone nutty enough to mug people in a graveyard.

We expected quite a crowd to attend this important religious holiday and were subsequently surprised to find ourselves whistling in the dark on a very lonely walk up the mile or so to the shrine. I'd been showing Mike how to read energy and we were having a lot of fun watching how some of the old, old family shrines oozed a menacing brownish energy rather like the fog in a grade-B British horror movie. I don't know in detail how Mike perceived some of this, but he jumped around quite a bit, looking over his shoulder while suppressing gibberish. It just looked like foggy energy to me, but then I'm used to having this so-called gift. I'd worked for it and no unexpected weirdness was going to spoil my walk, so we compared notes and hastened right along. No sense making closer inspection when we had a church service to attend. The next time a Zen monk warns me about protection I'm going to ask a whole bunch of questions (and not about the local crime rate).

When we arrived we were again surprised to find that the ten or twelve Americans outnumbered the Japanese in attendance. There was a small choir of chanters screaming rhythmically what sounded to me like "Turkey in the Straw" sung in Chinese. It must have been the intensity of their plea not the beauty of the call that attracted the spirit. As one group of chanters faltered from exhaustion, they would be replaced by alternative wailers.

It seemed to be working. The little shrine behind the big temple where Kobo Daishi's mummy was kept had a major energy form made up of lots of little sparkly lights that reminded me of the "Beam me up, Scotty!" effect on Star Trek. I decided that prudence required that I ignore it. Michael kept taking off his glasses and cleaning the lenses and putting them back on, then taking them off and cleaning them again. As a physician he is a very astute observer and does not trifle with observations that might question his credulity. Finally he says, "Do you see that weird light whizzing around?" *Folies á deux* confirmed, I shook my head, "Yeah, but I don't have the faintest idea what it is. Let's move right on out of here at the next break." I then blocked off his throat chakra, as I remembered reading somewhere that was supposed to protect one from psychic assaults (and it had worked for a couple of my students who liked to give each other headaches and nightmares), and we boogied.

The totally unexpected—even if harmless—sucks up a lot of energy just in the attention it requires. I still feel a little uncomfortable dealing with "The Undead." Particularly somebody else's. Mike and I are still good friends and are doing some fun papers together concerning death touch. He'll probably have to change his name so he can keep working. My reputation has already been ruined with reports like this.

I didn't realize this at first, but when you give someone energy, eventually it returns to you if the receiver no longer needs it or it just wants to visit Daddy for a while. You might not recognize the poor bedraggled little boogie when it shows up. The first time it happened I thought I was being attacked and sent it off with no praise at all for finding its way down the hall all by itself. The next time I was more gracious and curious and spent the night in joint study. After all, a loved one should not be abandoned regardless of where they've been or what they've been put up to. We all are capable of change even when we fall far short of expectations or the gentleness necessary to loving interchange at a higher level.

My first wife, anthropologist Martha Binford, had a wonderful childhood growing up among the Quechua Indians of Peru, as her father was William Howland Butler, a professional civil servant and ambassador to many countries in South America after World War I. Her mother was beloved by the Indians as a healer, and greatly feared by the rest of the family for her disgraceful sexual behavior. She claimed to be a high-level yogi and died as a remittance woman in Spain. Some of the stories Martha told me about her were verified by other members of the family. Her father was Surgeon General to India and the China Seas back in the days of gunboat diplomacy, and Martha's mother got to interact with some very strange people when she was growing up. This openness to esoteric phenomena led Martha to befriend a witch doctor or female shaman when she was doing her anthropological Ph.D. field research in Mozambique.

Martha attended a seance and tape-recorded it. When the spirit moved through the shaman her voice would change to a man's, and Martha said she spoke in a dialect of Zulu that was very old and no longer spoken by the Rjonga. She said the Zulu spirit was feeling rather shy because the old white spirit that was protecting her was different from anything it had ever seen before, and then it described her mother's father down to the old military medical uniform of the surgeon general. He was a very large man with a beard. Martha felt much safer in her studies after that conversation. Not speaking any of the above languages I can't verify what the tape said exactly but I think I can vouch for her honesty in translating. The drumming was similar to American Indian drumming popular with some of those studying shamanism these days, and the voice changed radically.

As you can see, my viewpoint on what I'm describing is pretty cross-cultural. Martha taught me to be a participant observer. You might say this report is a bit like what an anthropologist does but I am not interested in recording the visible history, just illuminating the hidden. Spirit is not just an attitude or something invoked by a pretty cheerleader. "To inspire" is not what a thrill it is to meet a personal hero. Our language is not without symbolic content. We have just elected to be familiar with the easier meanings of the words. The map is not the territory. The word may not be the meaning. If you can capture the meaning, you'll better understand kuji and juji.

The *musha shugyo* (solitary wandering of the Japanese hermit archetype) can be interpreted also as the journey within necessary to discover how your mind, body, and spirit really work. This can take many years depending on your diligence and knowledge and willingness to accept guidance in order to avoid damage. You are still on your own and have to do it by yourself. There are no teachers at this point; only your heart or inner light can sustain and guide you. If you want juji then you must seek out Hatsumi if you're following a ninja path. A high-level yogi or practitioner of chi kung may act as a helpful substitute. Jungian and Reichian psychotherapy can also provide some guidance, but you're still on your own.

Juji, according to Hatsumi, is more aligned with the mothering, female, or Wind aspects of energy—Yin, the absorbing—and if you like symbols, the dark tear on the Yin/Yang circle, which also is part of its opposite. Now we're talking androgyny, which is a little higher issue than gender. If you are going to "be all that you can be" there are energy exercises that open the mind to experiencing the universe from entirely different perspectives. I think these should be approached as if you were an exploring, intelligent child, as opposed to a warrior, warrior/priest, or mage. The perspective I've come to admire is more that of the sage. That may be just a by-product of my age and experience but it has led to the meeting of many remarkable men and a few women like Lee Bluesking or Shannon Kubiak who are also world-class martial artists.

The stronger spirit wins and knowledge is power. If your training is so limited that all you can do is march in a straight line smashing all before you, it's pretty evident that gaining the benefits of juji and kuji requires a long journey. Those whose only solution to difference is to murder the different in battle usually have limited options escalating far beyond normal perceptions of social intercourse. They tend to earn their destruction, be it losing the abilities they love due to age, arthritis, impotence, or the death-bringing sword in glorious battle, goaded on by spirits they should have learned to fear.

Chapter Seventeen

The Spider Prince

S TEPHEN HAYES HAS built a beautiful dojo and training center for his Kasumi-An, Nine Gates Institute in his hometown of Germantown, Ohio. I attended his seminar entitled Ninja Mind (May 4–5, 1991) and had a good time participating and watching him and his students. As usual I learned a lot of things and had some points clarified that I'd let slip. He led us through a series of mental reframing exercises drawn from the Mikkyo tradition that had immediate healing effects, presenting them in modern terms through physical exercises, meditations, dialogue, group process, and mini-lectures. It was a bit like attending an AHP convention except the students and teachers get to try to beat on and dodge each other.

Hayes is a good teacher and I've always been impressed by him. I had a chance to talk with some of his students and they were happy and busy working on their selves and preparing for their next physical test. The testing was public, and a board of black belts sat as judges of the students' taijutsu. Both men and women showed prowess and natural movement. Both those promoted and those who were not seemed to think the judgment fair and free of politics. I saw old friends from years back and some of the early black belts who I never got to know very well but can recognize. We seem to be aging gracefully.

I talked to one of the parents of a girl who had survived an attempted rape at a swimming pool. He had enrolled her in Steve and Rumiko's children's class. He was so pleased with the positive growth she was experiencing, and since the Kasumi-An training requires that parents attend with their offspring, he was learning too and getting a lot closer to his daughter. He said that like many girls who are victimized by rape when too young to know better, she was blaming herself and feeling guilt. She had lost her trust of men and adults as protectors and was much more fearful in general. (Not a life pattern that a responsible person would like to see developing in a daughter.) He said all that was turning around. He expressed the usual questioning of whether a child will ever really appreciate what they are being exposed to or realize the skills of their teachers.

Dennis Kinsalla was there. He's an actor who works out of Chicago. He showed me Steven Turnbull's book on ninjutsu, which was filled with beautiful old prints, historical descriptions, and lots of misinformation. The foreword by Hatsumi is priceless. Hatsumi quoted Takamatsu as saying you should go to original sources if you want to know history and pointed out that this would probably become the standard text on ninjutsu. Dennis had me look at the photograph of Turnbull and Hatsumi at the front of the book, as Hatsumi is not inscrutable to anyone who reads nonverbal behavior. It is easy to see which man feels he is in the presence of greatness. Hatsumi was practicing his Mona Lisa smile.

I borrowed the book to read in my hotel room that night, and one of the prints really caught my eye. It shows a Japanese prince identified as a ninja. The caption says "Prince so and so . . . planning an assassination." In the book's prose the ninja were identified as Chinese bandits and outlaws who had memorized Sun Tzu. Where does this Ninja Prince come from? (Ninja are nobles? Samurai weren't even considered nobles; they were managers of the royal holdings.) Hayes refers to ninja as freedom fighters; an even more accurate term might have been refugees who refused to be conquered, trapped on an island with their conquerors. The losers in a Japanese war are supposed to commit suicide. Warriors who are into Social Darwinism regardless of culture or age like the idea of "the winner takes all," as it simplifies the establishment of the New Order.

Taoists and Buddhists believe all life is sacred and our task on Earth is to create awareness or sentience. To take a life, even your own, is not following the Way. The ninja chose to live under the sword of the winners but moved into the mountains and away from the central government and established religion, which would have treated them as slaves and cowards. It is only normal that they would form a secret quasi-military vigilante group to protect their interests which would over time be demonized by the establishment.

A Japanese social anthropologist described Togakushi (I would translate the name in baby talk as The Straight Sword Mountain of the Loving Heart Knights) as the place "the wild people came to live and worship." Wild usually refers to animals we cannot tame. The place is a ski resort now, so the wild people are still drawn to the mountain. It's very beautiful up there and not easy to get to, even today. It is worth the trip.

The Spider Prince, as he was named in the picture, was garbed in green and gold. What do we know about the symbolic use of those colors? His hair was coiffed in the samurai manner but I don't know which clan, as I've never studied the hairstyles of the Japanese warriors. It gets a little crazier than vets and crewcuts.

The Spider Prince is pictured with an old scroll in his mouth that is tattered and stained. A ragged scroll is a Japanese artistic stylization that indicates internalizing knowledge that one is reluctant ever to use, as it is damaging to the user's very being if improperly applied. A scroll indicates a text that is written with such depth, clarity, and intent that one who reads it is immediately filled with new insights on his or her condition, regardless of the number of times read. It is not just memorization; it is transfer of training. Reading a scroll over and over has no effect, as the meaning will not sink in until you understand it. You only understand it through observation and behavior. Behind the prince is a huge, black spider with slavering venomous jaws and glistening eyes. Its size completely enshrouds the prince with shadow as a black aura. He looks frightened but determined. According to picture notes, the text of the scroll refers to the black mountain spider, probably a not-too-distant cousin of our black widow spider.

Now what can a prince, a man both bred and educated to care for the welfare of his defeated people, learn from studying a spider? Solomon, a king revered for his wisdom and songs for lovemaking, recommended that his people study ants. He had many wives and was said to commune with all of them, no matter how young and inexperienced or strange and exotic. As few people mentioned in the Bible are given the official designation of wise, it might be considered wisdom to develop some interest in Solomon's lifestyle.

Most warriors wishing to be known for their valor in battle study animals, as do sages—and ratrunners. Dr. N.R.F. Maier, my mentor, used to run *Norwegicus ratticus* instead of white mice. He ran the brown rats in size-to-size hedgerows or mazes to match them against the children of college professors. The brown rats kept up with or beat the kids to the prizes until the kids were around seven. Seven-year-olds or older usually could figure out the mazes quicker than the rats.

I was never certain if this was a comment on parenting skill or a demonstration of how swift and smart the rats were. He had one for a pet called Angel Face. There's a picture of it in an old *Life* magazine. It liked to ride around with him in his car, and his wife Ayesha told me, "The damned thing loved chocolates. You couldn't hide a box anywhere in the house that it couldn't get at it." Maier was the greatest American organizational consultant of his time. He liked problem-solving, as do rats, or we would have wiped them out long ago. The teenage mutant ninja turtles' sensei is a large rat. I've always liked monkeys. I was bitten by one as a child trying to pet the little savage. Study at a distance is fine by me as far as monkeys go. I read the primatologists.

Now go back and read the above description of the painting and commentary, thinking about it from the viewpoint of a humanistic psychologist who has had anthropological training and a Ph.D. in communication. Think of part of it as a riddle, part of it as a statement about the presenter. What am I saying between the lines? What are the deeper meanings? You've just been handed a mini-scroll. A scroll is supposed to be a work of art representing the accumulated skill of the master at a given point in time. Humor and trickery are respected characteristics of a ninja master.

I wonder what Norm did with the demographics on the kids? The master's thesis might be entitled "Interviews with the human beings who couldn't beat wild rats at solving mazes, and the tragedy of their further pursuit of a meaningful life: a longitudinal study."

A spider researcher might discover that insects outnumber humans in terms of diversity and number, and spiders are almost universally feared and disliked, yet thrive in practically every environment. The female vagina is perceived as a venomous, rotting spider to the insane across cultures. Why is this web-weaving creature sent by God to teach us? What can we learn from the black widow concerning the behavior of human beings?

We eat what we love. We kill what we love. We love who feeds us. Powerful women are dangerous. Make the dangerous beautiful. The powerful ones will kill you if they get pregnant. Birth control is a good idea if you want a powerful woman. Behind every good man is a better woman. If you don't want his children, get rid of him or cut his balls off. Rape prevention, too. We act to protect our genes. Be nice to your wife or she will be your death. Hell hath no fury like a woman scorned. There is a harsh wisdom worth pursuing our eight-legged teachers to learn.

How 'bout Daddy Longlegs? Balance. It has the deadliest poison but can't bite human beings. I've seen spiders that can walk on water and some that move along pretty well under it. I know the little rascals thrive all over the house, and you're continually dusting their webs above and below eye level. They are particularly good at establishing networks, yet they also toil alone. They hide in the still, dark, narrow ways. Some even seem to fly, as they use their webs for many tasks from communication to mobility as well as a trap for their prey. Even the big ones usually don't come charging out to greet you; they've learned caution right into their breeding. There's some poor Koga ninja I've seen on Japanese television who has poisoned himself with more than four hundred spider toxins. He has beaten calluses on his hands that jut out like knobs. He likes to climb the walls of the old palaces. He was some sort of engineer. His brand of spider knowledge has limited interest, as he confuses fear and love while seeking respect. His is the stereotypical ninja image. I can't recommend it but he seems happy. His nonverbals are a little odd, probably because of the poison. He looks the type to sweat it out rather than be humiliated by total evacuation. Spider venom is neurotoxic and affects how electricity is processed in the brain. His interpretation of Sun Tzu's references to the web of life don't conform to my idea of grace under pressure.

"Ichi" means one or the best in Japanese. (That is probably an indication of chi's place in the minds of those who formulated their mathematical system. That kind of pun and double entendre cannot be an accident.) Niten Ichiryu, Musashi's name for his "best school of the two swords" can also be translated as "body/mind heaven using the best chi." "Kunoichi" could be broken down and translated in baby talk as "the loving heart or stance is best." Kunoichi are spies of the ninja female variety for gathering intelligence. Women who practice ninjutsu are referred to as kunoichi. The spider way would be to send in your best first. Women are the better survivors. Women and children first. The lesson of the black widow indicates that a man's heart is below his stomach. Make the desirable feared and people will study what they practice.

Sun Tzu says treat your captured warriors well. Make the undesirable attractive. A traditional Japanese supervisor cares for his subordinates. A supervisor in a traditional organization will even act as a matchmaker if required. Arranged marriages are a universal trait of royal families. It usually results in some pretty spectacular inbreeding and blood diseases. The ninjas seem to prefer exogamous marriage or marrying out of the clans, differing from the xenophobia of the typical Japanese and materialism of European royals. Sun Tzu highly recommends the life of adventure on many levels.

An arranged marriage indicates a bond between families. It was often used in the West to prevent wars, as the grandparents tend to love their children's offspring even when it's hard to control their own. In warfare the beautiful kunoichi has an easy time reaching the beds of the leaders if they are far from home. Do not be aggressive; make the enemy come to you. A journey of a thousand miles begins with a first step. Taijutsu is defensive. It is drawn from the fighting styles of Chinese nobles and adventurers. There is even a spider kung fu which is associated with the emperor's teachers. Takamatsu said you have to follow the silk trail. The kunoichi is skilled in both the recognition and gathering of intelligence. She reports back along her network but being ninja has plenty of autonomy and options. In a man's world it is truly embarrassing to have your butt whipped by a girl, particularly one thought of as your wife or lover. Women in general appear very subservient in Japan. Most of the ninja women I've met were happy and articulate. We all know and care for Rumiko Hayes. She's a pretty woman from a country village in the mountains near the sea.

I had heard that Rumiko thoroughly thrashed Jack Hoban in a mock knife fight when he was teaching the knife fighting methods favored by the U.S. Marines, in which he was a captain. I've always fancied my knife work. I like a good match. I'd never been beaten. I wanted to try her out. In 1984, I cleverly managed to partner up with her when she was eight months pregnant. (I do not believe in giving away advantage.) She's a bright, cheerful spirit with soothing mannerisms. It's hard to believe she can tame demons, but Jack was a pretty hard boy. The moment I cut she had me stretched out in an arm bar using her rounded belly to pin my elbow. (Even the ninja fetus has potential to kill. That would make a great *Original Ninja* magazine headline.) This locked my arm and knife hand across her knees, forcing me to the earth; with both her hands free she dragged my 220 pounds as she walked duck-like, taking away my knife. Her spirited action convinced me that ninjutsu was an art of true self-protection that surpassed any physical training I had ever encountered. Her skills might be described as chiropractic. She pulled off this feat without even breathing hard and I took no damage while she knocked me about. She always refers to Hatsumi as Hatsumi-sensei. Many Americans think that she is Hatsumi's daughter. She's not but it seems a good idea to see her that way.

It was a treat to see her at the Ninja Mind seminar. Her skin was glowing with health, and I finally got to meet the daughter I may have frightened all those years ago. Both daughters were bright and cheerful, scrubbed and happy to see all their crazy uncles. One was joking about getting A's in recess to bolster her average. I showed Rumi the diploma Hatsumi had sent me. Her first words were "Ah. Hatsumi-sensei has sent you a shidoshi's license." Then she translated it for me. That took care of the idea that it would be fun to send me an official pass to a Tokyo brothel which started off "If you read Japanese don't laugh because he thinks...."

I hear a high-level American instructor is engaged to a Maramatsu clan girl. She was over as a translator for Hatsumi at the New Jersey Tai Kai. Pretty girl, funny sense of humor, and smart to handle the translation, which requires the ability to think esoterically in two languages as well as martial art codes. It's fun to hear how Hatsumi describes something in baby talk. English was not part of his studies. According to modern biolinguists, languages are learned best young as the brain is most flexible and there is a biological proclivity to acquire language that seems to kick in about two and may pretty well dry up by adolescence if not exercised.

People always sound foolish in a new language, particularly if they like to joke. I was never exposed to foreign languages until I was in high school. My French professor in college told me I was clever but hopeless, too late to learn a tonal artistic language like La Belle Langue Française. When I first saw the Dalai Lama in the early seventies, I made the mistake of not paying as much attention to his baby talk and listened more to his translator, who spoke my language with exceptional clarity. The message was essentially the same but the Dalai Lama exhibited a greater sense of humor. The other guy was showing off his language skills.

Hatsumi uses many illustrations drawn from the observation of nature. He has a lot of pets and walks them every night. The pets are gifts from students who don't realize that space is limited in Japan. I only have the faintest idea how he maintains the cardiovascular systems of his owl and turkey. Ben Franklin studied turkeys and thought they better represented Americans than eagles, now a threatened species. Merlin, the legendary advisor to King Arthur had a fondness for owls. Many of the observers of ninjutsu regard this as eccentricity. It looks like higher wisdom to me.

Sun Tzu's *Art of War* (which is also translated as *The Art of Strategy*) could also be translated as an "Art of Chi," particularly the sections dealing with adventure and intelligence gathering. R. L. Wing has done the best job of translating to date; if he were familiar with chi kung and the Go Dai he could have revealed another level hidden in code. It is my hope that his translation becomes the standard work. His feel for what is written is excellent. He's Chinese, bilingual, and an excellent writer of clarity. His subtitle for the work, "The World's Most Widely Read Manual of Skillful Negotiations and Lasting Influence," lets the astute reader realize he isn't referring to the Americans fighting their way into the bookstores so they can have this on their bookshelf right next to Kitty Kelley. He refers to the section associated with the spider prince as The Divine Web. He understands baby talk.

The story of Samson and Delilah is a classical example drawn from the Old Testament of the development of chi and fits nicely into our discussion of Spider Princes. His story is in the Book of Judges. Samson was a Judge of his people (a title having more to do with connection to God or exhibiting extremely violent creativity if you kick back and read the King James Version again), a rich kid and a great warrior who wore no armor and carried no weapons as the Philistines had captured and overrun Israel. (A similar situation to the Okinawans and ninja when overrun by samurai.) In one of his recorded battles he slew many of his enemies using a pick-up weapon, the jawbone of an ass. What else he did with that bone is really interesting. (Bone in Chinese medicine has many uses; some are said to be aphrodisiac. They might be interested in the properties of mule bones.)

Rather than dally with his own kind, Samson loved the women of his greatest enemy and his people's conqueror as a statement. In those days hair was thought to be a connection to the gods of the air. Then as today hair was also a mark of beauty as well as strength. (Taking someone's scalp is a little trick the French and British encouraged in the Indians of North America.) A woman of the enemy named Delilah conspired to capture him using lies, ties, and magic numbers. Even when he was being abused Samson enjoyed the game and would ignore her treachery and witchcraft as she was such a skilled lover. It was not his first folly with Philistine women.

The story is worth reading again now that you know some of the codes. Do you suppose there is a relationship between Nazarite and Nazarene? His heart was definitely below his stomach, not in his hair. But, he was a man of his time, and beliefs affect reality. We tend not to do what we don't think is possible.

He told her the secret of his strength was in his hair. It's a good thing he didn't think it was in his balls; that probably saved his life. She cut off his hair while he was sleeping off a drunk and probably drugged as well. (That's my version; he doesn't strike me as the type who would sleep that deeply over sex.) His enemies captured him easily as he thought he was weakened, because for him chi was a gift, not something developed. It just grew. If you've ever had a chi hangover the pain goes from the top of the head to the tips of the toes; when your whole body hurts and your mind is impaired it slows you down to normal.

The Philistines imprisoned this righteous man who thought of women as heifers when angry and never noticed his mother was smarter than his father (it's in the story), blinded him and put him to forced labor. The story goes they forgot to keep trimming his hair so it grew back so long and so strong that he was able to pull a temple down on those responsible for his humiliation. The reality of the tale might be that he had been sensory-deprived, had time to meditate, was mostly isolated, certainly celibate, somewhat starved, doing strong physical labor, in constant fear, and without his hair had to go into himself to find strength.

The Hindu, Oriental monks, and samurai who shave their hair are making a statement about their peaceful intentions and/or what aspect of God they serve. Only the highly skilled in spiritual matters or seekers of peace shave their heads. We in the West associate it with defeat and prostitution. Monks and holy men are known for their strength. It's more of a biker thing these days, but the emotional content is somewhat similar if wilder. The wise men knew we all serve more than one master.

When Samson needed all his strength he drew on all the sources available, even the gods of his beloved enemy. He was a Mensch, he liked animals and insects. He also understood endurance. Judges as a book puts some very dark behavior in a positive light. The term "judge" would include execution of action, as judges embodied the Law in Old Testament meaning. When I asked my daughter what she'd learned and remembered from the story of Samson she said, "Delilah cut off his hair so he wouldn't fool around." Linda thought he pulled down the tower of Babel. History is always being rewritten by the winners.

I think the story of Samson and the Spider Prince have some interesting correspondences, as does Musashi. We know little of what happened to the ancient ruling families of Japan who held the mountains. The archaeological evidence suggests that they were Chinese adventurers who had already cut a swath through Korea. Both ancient and modern stories suggest considerable exchange between the mountains of Japan and China. (Many Chinese masters say they studied with nameless Taoist masters on a mountain that they won't reveal.) Most martial arts combine like oil and water. Ninjutsu and the secret martial arts of the Chinese nobility flow together like honey and butter, to use a chi kung allusion. A close reading of Sun Tzu, a personal knowledge of the higher-level men and women who are members of Bujinkan as well as Chinese Arts, and a knowledge of art, language, medicine and history reveal a long-suffering noble face to this ancient and misunderstood art of spider princes and princesses surviving the death bringing sword of oppression. Living under the sword is a battle cry of the underground, where the sword over the heart indicates murder. The kanji is the same to my eye and indicates endurance that is heroic and worthy of study. The real thing is worth the journey. A follower of Sun Tzu starts the journey with one step.

I was asked to give a demo of ninjutsu to Mauck Elementary School in Hillsdale for the children's academic award day. Rumor was I was going to break flaming concrete blocks with my head. The kids were excited, the teachers weren't. I invited five or six young volunteers up on the stage. I spent about three minutes showing them how to do a simple wrist technique which throws people to the ground. I showed them how to roll and fall. We had a soft mat. I paired a small blond third-grade girl against a big-for-his-age, fifth-grade, red-headed boy who the teachers told me later was a bit of a bully. The little girl slammed him to the mat, jumped over his prone body, and ran off the stage back to her seat, grinning from ear to ear. He walked around shaking his wrist, trying to figure out what happened. I hadn't coached her beyond the basic technique. She understood ninjutsu and did the right thing. She knew he was dangerous. I gave her a bow. History can repeat itself in small ways.

Chapter Eighteen

Spirits—In Vino Veritas

SURPRISINGLY IN THIS age of Budweiser Light and Dry and unprecedented variety in ales, I occasionally have a student ask something like "But what does beer do? Why do people like something that tastes so bad?" Makes you just die to offer them a neat malt scotch like Lophraig or some twenty-year-old brandy. Talk about offended taste buds! You have to learn to look knowing and mutter, "It's an acquired taste. Took me years to discriminate. Wonderful bouquet. Slips right by the gag reflex. Smoooooth." My kids stayed away from the hard stuff as I never use mixers in the home. Let them find out about the sweet drinks after they've grown wary. It will be around. They are curious.

Human beings have been using alcohol for at least 25,000 years, primarily beer or similar beverages. The archaeological record is quite clear that almost all primitive societies used mind-altering substances. Even Neanderthals buried their dead with flowers and herbs, which strongly suggests a religious pharmacopoeia. Primatologists have told me that chimps will wait until the bananas are in a state of rotting fermentation, stake out and defend a tree, eat the bananas, get rip-roaring drunk, and often-times injure themselves seriously falling out of trees. As chimp doctors are rare on the ground, these drunks are often fatal, as the injuries make them more vulnerable to leopards.

My medical friends inform me that the body burns booze like any other food. The problem is the side effects. Side effects are both psychological, which will vary from individual to individual, and biological, which is somewhat easier to measure as body configurations aren't as difficult to quantify. We tend to measure what we can.

Many cultures have paid closer attention to the effects of diet, nutrition, and beverages than we have, particularly in regard to drugs and their effects. Did you know that alcohol in all of its many manifestations is considered a depressant, stimulant, and anodyne? Go get your dictionary and look up the last one. That's the one that will cause the troubles.

An anodyne releases the spirit, and that is what the addict pursues and often in his or her ignorance confuses with the stimulant or depressant effect. The trick is to sustain the spirit without becoming dependent upon the libation. It can be an aid to self-remembering, but the side effects are the gateway to hell. One has to be stronger than the spirit of the drug, and you must always be more interesting than its effect on your body.

The old word for alcoholic beverages was spirits. Indians referred to marijuana as "the benefactor." Tobacco was used for peace negotiations and in purification ceremonies. Hallucinogens were used for religious ceremonies, or for increasing psychic skills. All of these substances have receptors in the body and brain which relate to the release of endorphins and result in a mild, relaxed euphoria. Psychoneuroimmunology research indicates these internally produced natural substances are more potent than synthetic opiates and are by-products when physical and mental well-being predominate in people who have a positive and trusting viewpoint toward themselves and others. The pragmatic ninja viewpoint of raising children in a manner that provides and reinforces a positive viewpoint can be regarded as great wisdom when considering the biochemical reality of a happy individual.

Our ancestors used drugs but they were difficult to produce or were used in their natural state. Our contemporary proclivity for reducing a product to its most potent state is the equivalent of using sledgehammers to kill mosquitoes. Many modern medical practitioners pooh-pooh herbal remedies and homeopathic medicines, but an objective observer will not be swayed by a white coat.

All chemical addiction has a spiritual component, which if dealt with properly will free the addict. The use of psychoactive drugs to contact spirits is common in most low-technology societies and is seldom associated with addiction when used for this purpose. Practice usually allows the intelligent to discriminate between the dream and reality. Spiritual practice that is not mindful can also be addictive.

Tobacco was given to us by the American Indians. They used it primarily for peace negotiations. Indian warfare was up close and personal. You knew your enemy and his grandfather and cousins. American Indians, particularly the warrior societies, had some interesting ideas concerning bravery. It was not uncommon practice to humiliate and torture a captive to demonstrate your moral superiority. When enough of the young men had been killed off on both sides that conducting warfare began to affect the gene pool or economy, and mothers were getting angry, peace would be sought.

Now when you're going to sit down and negotiate for your friends, family, territory, and loved ones with someone who skinned your brother and then gave him to the women to play with, it helps to be clear-headed and take the long view. Hence let us smoke some of this brown stuff which tranquilizes the spirit but does not affect clarity of thought. They didn't walk around with a pack of twenty in their pocket to hit on every eight minutes, when the rush from the last one subsides. Hostile people tend to get on better with others when they smoke. That's why when some people quit smoking, their friends and relatives very quickly put temptation back in their path. It's called self-defense.

Women who smoke heavily during pregnancy will often have smaller and lighter-weight babies, which is associated with sudden infant death syndrome. Emphysema is one of the more unpleasant side effects of clogging the lungs with smoke. Cancer of the mouth, throat, and lungs is significantly correlated. The urine of heavy smokers is mutagenic; eventually that could result in cancers of the urinary and genital tracts. These are long-term side effects to be avoided. Meditating is a more beneficial means to obtain clarity of thought and calm, and the effects are permanent. However, rationality seldom subjugates desire. An Ethiopian wise man told me one time that smoking was a good way to train the breath. "If you can do it and still smoke. . . . " Often heavy smokers are not happy with their lives so they enjoy the tranquillity offered by tobacco and rationalize the dangers of addiction. Some of the people who come to me to quit smoking fall into that category. Most started when they were young, against the advice of their elders. Tobacco is more addictive than most synthetic drugs.

Alcohol reduces inhibitions, which is a subtle way of saying it weakens the superego, so the natural self can more easily emerge. If your natural self is relatively uncurried below the knees or not well socialized, it is probably wisdom to avoid the spirit known as demon rum. However, we've been using alcohol for a very long time to render events more convivial. (Remember the chimps.) Researchers interested in brain function say that alcohol breaks down the barriers between brain segments. Research indicates that a glass of wine taken twenty minutes before attempting to memorize something significantly correlates with retention. We learn better when our social inhibitors are weakened.

The problem is knowing when to back off. Dylan Thomas wrote some of his finest poetry when altered by alcohol, as did Shelley. Our consumer-oriented society encourages one to easily go beyond the stage where the anodyne is effective. Studies concerning longevity indicate that an ounce or two of alcohol a day correlates with long life. (We tend to save it up for the weekend.) Research also indicates that most of the positive effects of alcohol begin to deteriorate after blood alcohol reaches .06 on the drunkometer. That's two beers for most folks. Alcoholics die of dehydration. If you're going to drink, include plenty of water in your practice. Eight glasses a day seems to be the most frequently recommended amount of H_2O, twelve to sixteen if you're physically active. If your lips chap you need more water.

Just as the sermon should follow communion, so should some useful activity follow the ingestion of alcohol. The prudent man studies himself when his inhibitions are down. Some activities that are enhanced by lack of inhibition are thought, conversation, dance, and self-exploration. However, nobody enjoys a habitual drunk, particularly after they begin to confuse the feeling of power with real power.

Women who consume alcohol during pregnancy often have deformed or retarded babies. Alcohol damages sperm as well. Getting drunk to make a baby is not one of the better strategies. Often the children of parents who drink heavily or inappropriately will have attention deficiencies that result in lifetime problems concerning learning and the ability to hold a job. Crack cocaine does even more damage to brain functions. Many gamblers who lose their family fortunes become alcoholics. Hatsumi's father was a gambler who became an alcoholic. Hatsumi did not explore the effects of sake until quite late in life, remembering the example of his father. He has expressed regret that he never had the privilege of getting boiled with Takamatsu, who often offered him a drink.

Marijuana has a number of interesting effects, first and foremost being the reduction of short-term memory. That's why it is referred to in the colloquial as "dope." Loss of short-term memory forces one to pay attention to the immediate, which enhances how and what one feels. Being more aware of one's feelings is a definite enhancement to a number of activities in the short term. Appetite is enhanced, as are sensitivity and night vision. The anodyne effect is double-edged in that marijuana's receptors in the brain are on both the right and left sides, and the chemical makeup of THC is similar to what are considered female hormones. So with the smarter users you get creativity, and the more macho get to experience paranoia. Welcome to the wonderful world of women. If you're going to kick in the more intuitive side of your brain, which also processes feelings, you must remember that we feel before we think. Since most of us, particularly men, have had a lot of training in ignoring our emotions, finding them in charge can have interesting consequences. Particularly if your mind isn't too well disciplined and your memory not well trained. Short-term memory centers of the brain are not fully formed until after adolescence. If you are young and not too bright, just say no. A 1991 poll of high-level spiritual practitioners reported ninety-four percent using marijuana at some point in their quest for enlightenment. (Charles T. Tart, "Influences of previous psychedelic drug experiences on students of Tibetan Buddhism: a preliminary exploration," *The Journal of Transpersonal Psychology* 23, No. 2.)

Coca, the favored drug of those who live high above sea level, attaches to the brain and heart. It is primarily a stimulant to the heart, as well as a pain killer to the body and mild euphoric to the segments of the brain that reinforce reward-seeking behavior. A useful herb for an environment where even breathing is difficult. Its side effects are reinforcement of superego and delusions of grandeur. That's why it is the favored drug of those who are lost in the material world. Delusions of grandeur help you to like yourself when your existence is meaningless and your viewpoint negative. Of course, you're a winner because you can afford this substance and the other poor boobs are losers because they cannot. Users of cocaine, if they are not destroyed by their drug- induced violence and greed, often check out with heart attacks. One of the effects of cocaine allergy is severe vasoconstriction usually resulting in death. We seem to have forgotten that motto of the hippies as we moved to yuppies—Speed Kills. It's hard to work with the breath when your nose bleeds.

Anodynes can serve as an aid to meditative practice, but there is always the danger of addiction. The proper use of an anodyne is to memorize the desired state, push through the side effect, keep only what is useful, and use the rest for food. To do that requires strength of will and focus of intent beyond the capacities of most people unless they have developed their chi. Because they have no knowledge of how to use the released energy, they settle for the stimulant or depressant effect and are eventually overwhelmed by toxins.

Drugs are the fast food of enlightenment, as EST is the McDonald's of Buddhism. LSD, mescaline, and psilocybin can open doors to different realities, but when the drug wears off so does the induced state—if indeed the user is capable of perceiving the difference. To reference Tart's 1991 population again, psychedelic drugs were experimented with and seen as a positive aid to lucidity and clarity but were eventually rejected because of the tendency toward addiction to an easy source of luminosity. The wise learn to control the self with the self.

In terms of martial practice, one is much more likely to be involved in a fight when drinking—or a car wreck, or any other kind of self-destructive behavior that might emerge when our inhibitions are down and the id is up. One does silly things like falling asleep at sixty or seventy miles an hour, particularly when the id is an undisciplined, poorly raised child, not a seeker of joy. If you fancy yourself as a fighter, it's reasonable to find out what you can do under these conditions. It's a lot safer to find out with a friend at home or in the dojo than a bar where you have no idea what you may be facing in an impaired state. Particularly when you don't know your limits or have not learned how to burn through them, for which you always pay a price, as the anodyne is usually a toxin.

Meditation is the gentlest of anodynes and therefore the most subtle and pervasive. Loving and taking joy in what you do is another, and probably most powerful of all is being in love. Not just loving as in total acceptance of the other, but being in rapport chemically, electrically, and physically so that you merge with the loved one. It is incredibly energizing and nothing like being in heat, though of course that's part of it. That's why gurus get in trouble in the West. Our culture is much more repressed sexually than the East, so when people discover the power inherent in loving sexuality they tend to go overboard or in their ignorance create attachments that may not be beneficial. As the highest-level healing spirit requires androgyny, gender confusion may also result.

Those who advocate celibacy don't understand their own sexuality as part of the godhead. Celibacy can be seen as a sign of immaturity and a certain indicator that your teacher has missed the point, as enlightenment is powered by controlling sexual energy. Denial is not control, and control in this case is without effort. Without effort does not mean you don't have to study. It means you know what you're doing so well it appears effortless. Once again being relaxed is critical. Pounding away to orgasm has little to do with making love and less to sustaining the spirit. It is simply rapid behavioral response to a pleasurable stimulus.

Herbal remedies, particularly ginseng, can be anodynes. I've found ginseng particularly efficacious and recommend overdosing at first until you find what works best for you. The amount found in most teas is worthless. Capsules have worked best for me. Try two or three daily with lots of water for about a month. Medical research indicates that ginseng promotes homeostasis, enhances endurance, and maintains steady blood sugar and blood pressure levels. It appears to protect the heart from restriction of blood supply, protects the liver from damaging chemicals, and stimulates the immune system. The much-to-be-feared side effect in men seems to be a return to youthful erections, probably something to do with freeing up blood flow. I'll wager you'll like the effect if you're male and over forty.

I strongly recommend studying herbs, Chinese medicine, and homeopathic remedies. If you're sensitive to your body, you may find the results surprising. After my second divorce, a yogini friend of mine offered me the homeopathic remedy for healing grief, which I took condescendingly. To my great surprise I found myself weeping in a very short time. My tears had nothing to do with our conversation. Aside from the sudden onslaught of blubbering, I remember the evening as a lot of fun. Since then I've developed some faith through experimentation with Bach flower remedies as well.

As Aldous Huxley pointed out, the doors of perception are both subjective and universal. Anyone with common sense should be able to discover when to peak (peek?) and when to leap through their own curiosity and experience. The great sages always point to moderation, not excess, nor abstinence. Legal ramifications usually support common sense. The pursuit of enlightenment by a warrior is rare, not common in any sense of the word.

Refining attitudes to create a felt reality is part and parcel to Tibetan Buddhism as well as hoshinjutsu and ninpo. Assuming a particular attitude in or toward a situation can often speed the learning of behaviors as well as deepen empathy and understanding. Just realizing that you are listening to the perfect teacher because you are the perfect student in the perfect place with perfect friends to support your study helps you realize and focus on the fact that now is the perfect time to actually accept the higher teachings. This attitude creates a certain childlike expectancy and immediacy of wonder similar to the effect of the anodynes described above. It's a feeling to be cherished and is referred to as The Five Perfections. Try it out.

Chapter Nineteen

Strategies for a New Age

WE ARE MOVING into a new age. I think that after the Age of Reason, the Industrial Revolution, the Atomic Age, and the Information Revolution which resulted in the Electronic Village and world markets, we are ready for an Age of Creativity that will be and is already becoming an age of techno-magic. The break-up of the Soviet Union lowers the danger of world war and may be the beginning of a Pax Capitalista that will result in the sharing of ideas and periods of growth that will indeed create a new world order. If nothing else it indicates the real pauci-ty of thought from political scientists or the prediction capability of political economists.

Times are changing. A universal shift of consciousness is in progress. A global mind change will also be shadowed by a fevered retrenching of ultra-conservatives, but it must be remembered that change through action or atrophy, growth or dissolution, is the natural arena of the creative artist and leader. One does not lead to the past.

In *The Book of Five Rings,* Musashi gives nine basic rules or strategies for living well in war-torn medieval Japan that still work today. If you haven't read the *I Ching* or Book of Changes, you should. I have a friend who made a considerable fortune as a futurist using that book as a guide to policy decisions for some major corporations. There are also computer applications of the book that are quite useful such as "Synchronicity." There are people who actually consider me wise instead of foolish and asked me how I would improve on Musashi's list, so I consulted the *I Ching* and it said "Increase," "Arousal," and "The Creative." Given this acceptance by the divining spirits, here are my words of wisdom.

1. Never allow the concept that you have learned all there is to know about anything gain a foothold in your mind regardless of your achievements or recognition. Always regard yourself as a beginner and approach new challenges as an exploring child.

2. Passionately care for others and show your care by treating them with interest, respect, and love. Always be willing to make the first caring move. Love your enemy.

3. Be willing to learn from anyone or anything. Do not put your trust in secondary sources in any matter that directly affects you. Knowing without doing is not knowing.

4. In problem-solving always involve those closest to the problem in the building of a solution. Get to the "we," as acceptance is necessary to quality. Always take time to discover the probable downstream effects of implementation. To quote Richard Weaver, an admirable rhetorician, "Ideas have consequences." Continuous improvement leads to better changes than embracing a past that does not exist.

5. Both the best and worst of people yearn to love and be loved and if given the opportunity would make a positive difference in the world. Be helpful and kind.

6. Study yourself as well as others and why you and they feel and care about the goals you (and they) pursue to develop staying power as well as trust. Do not waste your essence in a relationship where there is no caring. Learn to trust your gut, which isn't too far from following your bliss and helps you avoid the bitter taste of defeat.

7. Continually expand your awareness of your connectedness to others. Everything in the natural and material world is con-

nected in never-ceasing, ever-changing interactions and interdependencies. Be part of that, as the disconnections are illusions. Take every opportunity to become more open, aware, and challenged.

8. Understand that when you move, you move as a whole and are contributing to change by how you act and think. Put meaning, purpose, and passion into everything that you do. Be willing to sacrifice, to take risks, or to humble yourself to achieve a clear, concrete result. Modesty is the greatest of virtues. Censure yourself, never another. Have fun but don't harm. Internalize the Shaolin Dictums.

9. If you follow your bliss, allowing time for peaceful contemplation, and remember the ancient dictum that "defense is moral and offense often leads to disgrace," the Way of the Warrior/Artist/Sage will in the end be seen as profitable as any other form of sincere scholarship. Sincere scholarship seldom pays well until all other avenues have reported failure. The sweet taste of fortune is both spiritual and physical when the emphasis is on learned taste and the fortune is earned. The Zen Buddha of the Ten Pictures rides the ox to the marketplace.

I have had a great deal of fun studying strategy or combatic martial arts and have through these studies met very interesting people. There is an old Special Forces recruiting joke that goes, "Join Special Forces; Travel to Faraway Lands; Study Exotic Cultures; Learn New Languages; Meet Exciting and Interesting People (all at government expense) and Kill Them." Sun Tzu says, "It is only when you are a thousand miles from home that you will find the value of your most basic skills." Your most basic skills as a human being are to learn and to build relationships. We are ascended from social animals. An adventurer in the realms of strangers must be able to be perceived as valuable on some other basis than language, technical skills, or formal knowledge.

Sun Tzu's Divine Web of the adventurer and reincarnation has implications for vengeance and reciprocity as well as forgiveness. I sometimes find it difficult to maintain gentility when training with my friends in the martial arts. Those who need a healing spiritual practice the most seem to be running hardest in the direction of fear and power. I suspect they have unwittingly selected the "school sent by the nine demon gods." Some need a vision of Hell to appreciate Heaven's Way.

The world is changing and it appears that the environment requires some heroic consideration. I have found myself regarding the farming methods of the Amish with much greater respect of late. There seems to be a different cycle of reincarnation that favors greater understanding between Kipling's severed East and West. On the darker side, the decimation of Third World populations and the urban ignorant by poverty, drugs, HIV, and other smart viruses to come will increasingly tax the medical systems of the elite as well as confound the dreams of the careless and unlucky. The urge to religion is universal and healthy in terms of lower associated medical symptoms, even though the correlation between IQ and strong religious belief is significantly negative. The relation to health, however, is positive when compared to controls. My own experience of linking religious types to various neuroses may derive from a limited sample that has been taught to fear God and sexuality and see their religion as exclusive. There is certainly much better esoteric information available today than in any previous age. The scholarship and research published in the last ten years are astonishing. The books I recommend in the Bibliography for Inner Adventurers also have some of my brighter students' heartfelt approval. Even the charlatans are having to learn that the ignorant have been exposed to the scientific method and would like to see some replication of quality results before buying the product.

As more scientific seekers publish their own experiences rather than point at the wisdom of the elders for direction, we seem to be experiencing a "hundred monkeys effect" but it may well be information reformation and regression to the norm. People seem to be finally recognizing that human commonalities are far more important than the differences. Hatsumi, after he met me for the first time sent me a watercolor of Da Mo, the Bodhidharma and the founder of Zen who is credited with revolutionizing the martial arts as taught at the Shaolin Temple. The inscription was translated for me by a young Japanese exchange student who interpreted what he had written as "Constants Don't Surprise" for the symbol of ninjutsu, which is the kanji for sword over the kanji for heart, which also can be translated as endurance or following the way even when under duress. The rest of the poetic inscription was "The bear's treasure is joy and pleasure."

The above little list is my strategy for enjoying the newest age, as nine directed by a unique perspective leads to zero. There is nothing in this list that is not supported by scientific research in psychology, anthropology, and sociology. William James, the famous American psychologist, posited that we feel before we think, and there is considerable evidence to support that hypothesis. The subconscious is the seat of feelings, and if you follow the directions in chapter five you will learn how to link the emotions to the mind through meditation. The ancients called this practice Heaven's Way, and it results in the dissolution of fear, which enhances all other activities in life. It must be remembered that you shape the world you live in by your regard, and by opening yourself to complete experience you may find many surprising things that most other people will miss. This process will change you. It will change how you regard the world and others; it may even put a little magic and passion into your life if you follow the clues concerning weird science.

We all change, as does our environment and society. Humans are unique in that we can control and create those changes. Real change is seldom an act of instant conversion. A changed mind that is not followed by behavior has not reached into the true self. We can all work on ourselves and each other to make our lives more enjoyable and better, or we can be swept along by fads, worn down by indifference, and live in ignorance. The choice is always yours, but to paraphrase a wise and ancient Greek, "The unexamined life is not worth living. Know thyself!"

Chapter Twenty

What Good Is Enlightenment?

I N "THE KUNDALINI EXPERIENCE" I describe what the great awakening feels like, and in "the Godan Test" what the lesser awakening feels like in terms of sensitivity. In chi kung as well as Taoist esoteric yoga, these are referred to as the *greater and lesser kan and li*. In religious traditions enlightenment is associated with sainthood, or being in tune with (called by) God. In military traditions it's associated with invincibility in warfare and the use of superior strategy, as in Joan of Arc or Sun Tzu. In art and science it manifests as creativity. In yoga an enlightened master manifests the will of God through self-development. In common parlance enlightenment is referred to as being intuitive and usually thought of as an on-again, off-again experience related to luck. In chi kung it is considered a biological enhancement of natural proclivities and is permanent if the practitioner is careful and knowledgeable. Historically enlightenment is considered quite rare.

The technology for awakening intuition has been with us for centuries, but few seem to be willing to take on the challenge of integrating the mind, body, and spirit, as it requires concentration and very few seem capable of hanging in for longer than twenty minutes regardless of the importance of the topic. It does require an adventurer's heart, and the voyage is made alone regardless of who shares your journey. It could be described as the resurrection of the body. The end point is being born again or zero, and a viewpoint regarding life that is held by very few and could be regarded as delusions of grandeur or controlled paranoia were it not for the recognition that this is or should be anyone's birthright. Fearing God is the harshest way of saying Respect Yourself.

The thinking style of the enlightened is very relaxed and conversational, like a good story-teller, but the linkage of ideas is much more circular and nonordinary. The ideas themselves seem to come best from observation. The trait of empathy—which for males is usually hard-won learned behavior—seems to extend to all of nature. It's not sympathy but understanding how people or animals and sometimes plants and insects feel. It is usually referred to as knowing.

Sensitivity to how one's body is functioning is greatly enhanced for the more enlightened. One can feel the intestines working and sense the movement of energy and blood as well as control the rate of the heart. When a joint begins to slip out of place, you can often correct it by simply adjusting your posture. It is the same with a thought. Pain is controlled. The eyes see farther into the ultraviolet spectrum, and night vision returns if you've lost it. Middle-age astigmatism is corrected to some extent. The body's temperature drops to a range between 94.2 and 97.2 degrees Fahrenheit and often feels cool to the touch of others, but there is no sensation of chill to you except when you're cruising in the lower ranges. Being cool seems to have a biological consequence as do ideas. You are much more aware of the subtle energy fields surrounding yourself and others, and with practice and experience can discriminate differences that seem to be meaningful. To others you may feel warm or neutral due to energy rather than temperature. Fear of death and other inevitable occurrences evaporates. There is an acceptance of self that does not require external reinforcement.

Handedness becomes an option with sometimes amusing results. (This may also account for tantrism being called the left-handed way.) Most of the time the mind is silent and observes with no commentary. The immune system seems to be strengthened as healing time is shortened, colds become rare and of short duration, and the lower blood pressure and anal squeezing eliminate annoyances like hemorrhoids. Cuts heal quickly. What the long-term benefits of this change in a modern, free-enterprise society can be, I've no real idea. We seem to reward a blinder ambition.

We like to have goals. We like to know where we are going. The enlightened have no personal spiritual goals beyond deepening their experience, as enlightenment is the end product of the spiritual path. Some seem to attract the attention of the Web of Life and become guardians of the environment, reaping cosmic rewards. A few teach, and those who attempt to follow their guidance and fail find religions for their solace. The enlightened can tolerate no falsehood in themselves. In others, it's their problem to solve. From a religious viewpoint the behavior is usually regarded as saintly, and some rather odd people have been designated saints from a psychological perspective. From the churches' perspective, extreme examples are still examples of possibility and should be shown compassion. Some of Catholicism's choices are perverse and funny riddles. Protestants don't recognize saints but seem easily distracted by and willing to pay for uninformed hypocritical entertainment, as TV ministries like Roberts, Graham, Falwell, Tilton, and the Bakkers indicate.

In business, the enlightened owner provides challenging work so that continuous repetition does not dull the minds of his workforce. He or she encourages problem solving and creativity so that the organization can react to the marketplace. He studies the trends and tries to be ready for the future. He expects his people to educate themselves and provides time and opportunity so that they can improve their position in life through material reward or personal growth. He attempts to maintain a balance or a mix of rewards and products. He protects the econiche, which continually is endangered. He cherishes autonomy and creativity. He maintains excellent relations with his consumers and suppliers. He adapts to change and sometimes leads the charge when change is necessary. He is concerned with the quality and reputation of his product. He understands the meaning of service and synergy.

An enlightened artist is concerned with showing what is before the eye in a new way, so he or she is not concerned with convention or fashion once they've proven their expertise. Art is always personalized, and that which is recognized is imitated. Most artists who forge new paths or depart too far from the mainstream are not rewarded in their lifetimes. All true artists are concerned with mastery of their material. Great artists or masters (or mistresses) are adventurers who move out of their fields and expose themselves to other forms of knowledge which they then use to modify their own work or bring new insights to cross-fertilize. Their performance in the new area may be met with derision, but as they've proved their endurance in one area, it's usually not long before they acquire the necessary new skills. The Nobel Prize winner in one field should be given a polite listen when discussing another field.

The more information, interests, and skills artists acquire, the easier and more fluid the process of creation becomes. An artist may emerge in any occupation where there is freedom to experiment and opportunity to problem-solve or personalize change. America is a land of mini-artists who specialized too early or quit because they expected mastery to come sooner. Many decide to follow financial reward. Free enterprise is a wonderful concept that can both foster and destroy creativity. Art is the cradle of invention. War is the mother. Surviving takes both endurance and creativity.

The enlightened martial artist is concerned with defense and retaliation as a preventative therapy. Ambush and attack is the way of the bandit and the materialist and if used against an unintelligent enemy usually works. Really dumb or desperate people go toe to toe and slug it out. An enemy tries to harm you. War is the product of failed diplomacy. It is the rapacious consequence of greed.

A skilled strategist has many responses and can escalate or withdraw as necessary. Taking your best shot can be telling a joke, or walking away, or setting a trap. The samurai maxim "the best sword is never drawn" does not mean that it cannot be used. It refers to the mind and spine of an upright individual. A real master can read your heart, and show you how to attain peace. Worthwhile study if structured properly results in transfer of training. All of the high-level ninjas are working at seeing the light. The bad ninjas are disappearing. They're aging prematurely, as God needs fertilizer. As the training intensifies the ability to read others, the attitudes of your teacher may drive you to find another more to your liking.

Since Kevin Millis describes me as being from Mars, let me share with you what a Martian who is a human being feels like. I do not perceive myself as having any knowledge that anyone else can't have if they're willing to take the abuse and endure some risks. Divorce, financial ups and downs, chi-sickness and suffering should not be part of your quest but they can happen when you're not gonna quit till you get it, and you only have so much time because your experience has taught you this place can be hell. Enlightenment's at least a three-year process if you know what you're doing, but the short course can be very high-risk. It takes a lot longer as a part-time job and requires more than one day a week to accomplish or sustain. It's a lifetime project, as once the mind begins to move it wants to keep going.

Feeling the mind at work is almost orgasmic. It's very pleasant when the words and ideas just flow out of you. It's a mental side effect of taijutsu and meditation, as they both stimulate the spine and brain. Because you're more in tune with your body, you can feel disease or sore muscles as they start and often can dispel them before they hinder your movement. Adjusting the spine becomes very important, and when the back is out you can feel the drop in immune system efficiency. There is something to the Alexander Method and chiropractic. Pain is remembered, accepted as part of learning, and categorized as needed. There is no confusion once experienced between lust, love, and sexuality, though all are felt.

When you are relaxed—without fear but still able to use your adrenals—the mind integrates with and accesses subconscious memory. Subconscious memory seems to include some very surprising and curious talents. Physical sensitivity is greatly enhanced as well as balance and flexibility. There is a feeling of connectedness that is bioelectrical and when used enough to trust is never wrong. Entering someone else's electrical field gives you useful information if you remember yourself. It is very difficult to remember you can do this, as there is no social reinforcement for the skill. Dreaming can become a waking function as the subconscious makes the id's contribution to observed phenomena (visions and hallucinations are better accepted with equanimity if you are in a public place).

When you use your total self to look at something or someone, some insights will be visual as well as mental and physical feelings; these sensations often arrive in the dark as mini-hallucinations but are information if you've the knowledge to interpret and use them. In the old days it was consulting the Muses. Probably the verb "amuse" is related. It seems like great fun to me. It feels like the way we're "spozed to be." I think of it as awakening the sixth sense; a yogi would perceive it as union with the inner god that allows communion with the eternal spirit. A Buddhist might regard it as an evolutionary guide toward sentience. When you are self-remembering, it means you are fully aware of how you are processing information all the way down to your cells. You tend to be very much attached to the present reality. The past feeds you and the future awaits your endeavor. Some of your feelings can be very disturbing, but you have the choice on how to react to the bad news.

Salvation cannot be bought. A Christian might say you must save yourself. Enlightenment is not an intellectual position but a biological reality that is attained through work. It's like lifting weights or getting a degree. It requires self study, concentration, and time. It is only after the awakening that the process becomes natural and without effort.

The American Indians thought that creative people or those whose minds could move were bird people. They were excellent observers of nature. What can we learn from the common blackbird? Birds exhibit continual movement and high-burning metabolisms. They must continually search for sustenance and do not exhibit much territoriality. They have signals and warn each other of danger. They sing for their own enjoyment and probably entertain each other. They recognize hierarchy when feeding. They don't seem to have much short-term memory but can learn through repetition and reinforcement. Some migrate over vast distances. They enjoy acrobatics.

I was sitting on my back porch one day when a red squirrel dragging a very small nest ran around the corner of the house. It was pursue1 by a small starling. The starling would open up its wings to appear bigger and danced screaming at the squirrel, which was twice its size. The squirrel, seeing it was going to be cornered by the walls of the porch, scampered like a furred tree rat and leapt into the neighbor's pine. The starling's friends arrived and proceeded to throw themselves screaming at the squirrel, who was running up and down limbs trying to avoid their dive bombing. Two robins and a sparrow joined the fray. There was another nest in that tree. Birds of different species will join with each other to defend against a common enemy. The squirrel finally leapt from a limb about eighteen feet up, having seen the dangerous as attractive, and hit the ground hard. Scrambling in fear, it took off clumsily for the maple tree in the front yard as the small cloud of birds pursued like WWI biplanes or the X wings in *Star Wars* after a fleeing target. Reminded me of the Iraqis heading for the last bridge out of Kuwait. Sun Tzu recommends leaving an obvious exit for your enemy. Schwartzkopf showed how to close it.

I've seen songbirds go after hawks, crows, and owls who will eat meat of their own kind in order to feed their appetites. The predator birds are usually more territorial, mostly solitary, and do not sing. The owl is a creature of the night, having great nocturnal vision, acute hearing, and silent flight, giving it the ability to hunt in both trees and plain. The crow is said to be of great intelligence and far-sighted. It can be taught to talk like the long-lived parrots, only more quickly if you split the tongue. When our Red Brothers say a person speaks with forked tongue it can also mean the person is not true to his nature. Crows perceive man as dangerous to their species and give us a wide berth except at harvest time or when we appear to be unarmed. When you hunt you seldom get more than one crow unless you have a silent weapon or exceptional skill. Songbirds eat grain and insects. As do the bushmen. Carrion birds will show you death.

Mostly the bird people served as advisors or peace chiefs. Chief Joseph kept over five divisions of U.S. Cavalry including Buffalo Soldiers continually in the field with hit-and-run raids using less than twenty men while escorting his people's attempted escape to Canada. Tengu are birds. The tops of totem poles are often birds.

Teachings by tengu to samurai were preserved as scrolls even though few seemed to understand them. Even mastering one of the tengu's techniques was usually enough to protect you from the average attack. The message seems the same. "You're not meant for this. Only good people should be training with swords. Get out of it. I even have to beat you up to show you this simple stuff. You don't know how to think or act. You're not a pimple on the butt of a real swordsman, but these techniques will probably save your life considering the opposition." The tengu emphasized a morality for the use of the sword and discussed it as a weapon of defense. Tengu were not proud of their skill at arms and discussed swordmanship as a last resort, a necessary consequence of dealing with men. I suspect the legendary tengu of being teachers of the soft budo of Osaka and Kyoto. There is a direct mythological connection to the ninja. They were overrun, but never defeated, rather like the Seminole Indians of Florida.

Even today we demonize our enemies. When the law is breaking down and the people and politicians are exhibiting a mean spirit, those that exercise their freedom to learn self-protection seem the more survival-oriented to me. We still can learn from the birds. Survival can be pretty comfortable if you're intelligent about it. The great mother can tame demons and get them going in productive directions—protection of home and Momma and cleaning up the neighborhood—in subtle but effective ways requiring the aid of the residents. I prefer making the attractive dangerous. Life has given me the other training. Endurance is a path to enlightenment.

There is a ninja scroll on how you can tell the time by how the cat's eye normally dilates. I wonder what else it says about them. (The hand claws are pretty interesting. Ichimunji is a better cat stance.) I've seen this cat's eye chart reproduced in a number of books and I always thought it was a joke. If scrolls were kept by masters on many topics, a family of masters going back eight hundred years and more like the Togakure Ryu would probably be worth studying and learning new languages or very old ones. Takamatsu left pretty broad hints it extends back a lot farther. Sun Tzu says the learning doesn't really start until you're a thousand miles from home and you have to rely on your basic principles. Feelings are pretty basic.

If my conjectures are on target, the ninjas are correcting the way martial arts are taught and discussed and have every right to. Hatsumi has said on more than one occasion that ninjutsu owes the Chinese. He dressed up in Chinese robes and showed weapon techniques. Some of the male figures in the old ninja scroll drawings are wearing Chinese costumes in the Quest videos. He chose to show that for a reason. If this is the old snake brain functioning, it seems able to discern the light from the dark on a multitude of levels. Anthropomorphizing is considered to be bad science but my feeling is it can be intelligently applied to reality. In real science as well as combatic martial arts we practice skepticism and humility. In psychology, which gets off track from time to time, we say, "The rat is always right." Enlightenment seems to be recognition that all things are connected through love and intelligence. The shaman's viewpoint is reflected in the Book of Job. Chapter thirteen offers, "But ask now the beasts, and they shall teach thee; and the fowls of the air, and they shall tell thee: Or speak to the earth, and it shall teach thee; and the fishes of the sea shall declare unto thee." Keep going. Keep playing.

Annotated Bibliography
for the Inner Adventurer

This bibliography is designed to support *Path Notes of an American Ninja Master*. It is also the recommended reading list for the fourth-degree black belt in hoshinjutsu. I urge you, the reader, to buy and read the books in the blocs in which they're presented. Each book is representative of a classic position and is the best of its type in my opinion. If read in tandem, these books present a series of ideas that interweave to provide a unique understanding of the topic that will be different from the authors' and mine, but of particular use and benefit to you. Try it out and see. I'll wager you'll have as much fun as I did with a quarter of the effort.

The first two or three books in each section are the most important. There is no particular order for your perusal. The prudent individual builds his or her own library and supports the one in the local community. Reading is one of the universal skills of leadership. If Ben Franklin were around today, he'd say, "A book on line saves time."

Internal Energy

Dr. Yang Jwing-Ming. *The Root of Chinese Chi Kung: The Secrets of Chi Kung Training*. Jamaica Plain, Mass.: Yang Martial Arts Assn., 1989. Excellent text for explaining many of the consequences and side effects of learning to breathe and exercise internal energy or chi. Scientifically and experientially based, and only refers to the ancients for additional descriptions. Does show some energy applications for the martial artist that complement the healing art.

Mantak Chia. *Awaken Healing Energy Through the Tao.* Aurora Press, 1983. Written as clear, logical, and practical medical descriptions that encompass the physiological and spiritual practices for awakening and circulating chi. This is the basic book and contains practically all you'll ever need to know. Mantak Chia also has a valuable series of books relating to various other aspects of Taoist esoteric yoga, sexual practice, and nei kung published through Healing Tao, 2 Creskill Place, Huntington, New York 11743.

Ajit Mookerjee. *Kundalini: The Arousal of the Inner Energy.* Rochester, Vermont: Destiny Books, 1986. Describes the core experience of Tantra and relates it to the opening of chakras; provides both modern illustrations and ancient commentaries. An excellent overview and worth comparing to the Taoist cosmology.

Gopi Krishna. *Kundalini: The Evolutionary Energy in Man.* Boston and London: Shambhala, 1971. Describes the effects and personal experiences of an Indian gentleman who went through the kundalini with no real prior training or expectations beyond curiosity and rudimentary meditative practice. It nearly killed him and is a great cautionary tale as well as an accurate description. It should be read by anyone who wants to follow in the steps of their ancestors. Hillman's Jungian analysis of the experience widely misses the reality of being touched by the goddess.

Sexual Practice

Mantak Chia and Maneewan Chia. *Healing Love Through the Tao: Cultivating Female Sexual Energy.* Huntington, New York: Healing Tao Books, 1986. Absolutely the best book for women. Never give this to any female with whom you are intimate if you haven't finished your own work. You'll never catch up if she catches on. The ladies learn this stuff more quickly and easily than men because of the structure of the corpus colossum. They've one for male sexual practice called *Taoist Secrets of Love: Cultivating Male Sexual Energy.* New York: Aurora Press, 1986. You should read both.

Dr. Stephen T. Chang. *The Tao of Sexology: The Book of Infinite Wisdom.* San Francisco: Tao Publishing, 1988. Combines Chinese medicine and sex therapy in unexpected but beneficial ways. Easy to read and experiment with. Discussion of "million dollar point" is invaluable. However, his discussion of strengthening the immune system to cancel out virus-related infections is not supported by my experience nor observation of others.

Nik Douglas and Penny Slinger. *Sexual Secrets: The Alchemy of Ecstasy.* New York: Destiny Books, 1979. A wonderful book. Provides cross-cultural tantric practice as well as tips for getting into the attitudes of the gods. Must be read—though looking at the pictures will provide for hours of experimentation. Referred to in code by those in the know as The Big Red Book. The most practical and useful discussion of higher tantric practice I've ever found and I read a lot. No home library is complete without it if you are trying to understand Eastern religion, sexuality, and culture. Margo Anand's *The Art of Sexual Ecstasy* (Tarcher, 1990) provides modern application of these ancient principles for the beginning Westerner.

Dr. Alan P. Brauer and Donna Brauer. *E.S.O., The New Promise of Pleasure for Couples in Love: Extended Sexual Orgasm (an illustrated guide).* New York: Warner Books, 1983. It's fun to see what a bright young couple can figure out to do with sexual organs and a Western medical background. Go scientific method!

Gregory J. P. Godek. *1001 Ways To Be Romantic.* Weymouth, Mass.: Casablanca Press, 1991. This is my major failing in life. A little bit of this goes a long way. If you want to preserve a relationship or create one, let Godek be your guide. It's never too late. This book is a heartbreaker if you haven't a clue. My ex gave it to me in hopes I would reform. It's a frightening mirror. I've seen women burst into tears when reading it. The marriage you save may be your own.

Philosophy and Strategy

Miyamoto Musashi. *The Book of Five Rings.* Woodstock, N.Y.: Over-look Press, 1974. There is also a Bantam translation that is very good. The Japanese consider this the equivalent of a Gospel or Veda. It is a guide for the individual warrior and contains many useful techniques for disposing of swordsmen.

Sun Tzu. *The Art of War.* Any number of translators. I like R. L. Wing's *The Art of Strategy.* New York: Dolphin/Doubleday, 1988. The guide book for Chinese bandits and inner adventurers everywhere. Like go is to chess, Sun Tzu is to Clauswitz. Avoidance of conflict is the basis of all strategies, leading to eventual total and permanent victory.

Lao Tzu. *Tao Te Ching.* Aside from the Bible, the most translated book ever written. Once again, I'll support R. L. Wing's translation, *The Tao of Power: Lao Tzu's Classic Guide to Leadership, Influence and Excellence.* New York: Dolphin/Doubleday, 1986. There is no better prescription for skilled leadership than this subtle and marvelous guide to influencing others.

Lex Hixon. *Coming Home: The Experience of Enlightenment in Sacred Traditions.* Los Angeles: Tarcher, 1989. Ken Wilber thinks this is the best introductory work on the world's great mystical traditions. Hixon's presentation is unusually clear and easy to read. He moves from ancient tradition to contemporary practice with a knowing skill. This book is more useful for the beginner than John White's *What is Enlightenment.*

The Encyclopedia of Eastern Philosophy and Religion/Buddhism, Taoism, Zen, Hinduism: A Complete Survey of the Teachers, Traditions, and Literature of Asian Wisdom. Boston: Shambhala Publications, 1989. Tells you what the words mean, who the people were, and what important things they said. A helpful text when you are reading and people use esoteric language to demonstrate they've been East or talked to a guru who didn't know English words for his or her practice. (Sometimes there aren't any. Salvation or "being cool" really isn't the equivalent of satori or sammadhi.)

Dr. Christopher M. Bache. *Life Cycles: Reincarnation and the Web of Life.* New York: Paragon House, 1990. The last two chapters are brilliant and the rest of the book held my attention. The Web of Life and discussion of Sheldrake's field theory had me moving my lips. This is a very useful book as an interpretation of Sun Tzu's commentary on the Divine Web.

Warren Bennis. *On Becoming a Leader.* New York: Addison Wesley Publishing, 1989. A guide to modern leadership in organizations. Research-based and well written. if you are going to be a leader in the field of martial arts or just an excellent teacher of the way, this book will provide information that is just as useful as the more traditional Oriental texts concerning strategy and leadership.

Dr. Mihaly Csikszentmihalyi. *Flow: The Psychology of Optimal Experience.* New York: Harper and Row, 1990. A guide to the inner experiences that make life worthwhile. Psychological support for the Zen experience. He even cites ninjutsu as a possible route to physical liberation. Interesting book if you're pedantic or skeptical enough to need a totally Western viewpoint. He tends to squeeze the juice out of the lemons.

Herbert Silberer. *Hidden Symbolism of Alchemy and the Occult Arts.* New York: Dover Publications, 1928. Also J.C. Cooper's *An Illustrated Encyclopedia of Traditional Symbols.* New York: Thames and Hudson, 1987. Cooper explains all kinds of things if you haven't figured out that there is a basis to magic that is rather weird science. A knowledge of symbols becomes very important when you begin to visualize and communicate telepathically. Silberer's book is quite old and way ahead of his time. He was probably burned on a stake. He translates some old German alchemical texts and then performs a Freudian interpretation that is quite good.

Personal Health and Well Being

Bob Anderson. *Stretching.* Bolinas, Calif.: Shelter Publications, 1980. Stretching is necessary for the body's ability to process higher energy. This fun book of stretches is very helpful. If you want to be very knowledgeable, combine this with the analysis of asanas you get monthly in the popular magazine *Yoga Journal* and that will provide all the exercises you need.

Shizuto Masanuga with Wataru Ohashi. *Zen Shiatsu: How to Harmonize Yin and Yang for Better Health.* Tokyo, Japan: Japan Publications, Inc., 1977. People keep stealing my shiatsu books, and once you start experimenting with the techniques you'll understand why. Shiatsu becomes particularly interesting once you've developed chi kung.

The Editors of *Prevention Magazine* and The Center for Positive Living. *Positive Living and Health: The Complete Guide to Brain/Body Healing and Mental Empowerment.* Emmaus, Pa.: Rodale Press, 1990. The editors overstate their case, but this book is full of useful information and handy tips. All the health-oriented books from Rodale Press are excellent sources for the independent investigator.

Edward Bach, M.D., and F.J. Wheeler, M.D., *The Bach Flower Remedies.* New Canaan, Ct.: Keats Health Classic, 1979. You have to try these things. You should also learn about homeopathic medicine. I know of few martial artists that don't respect chiropractors and massage therapists, for that matter.

Ted Kaptchuk and Michael Croucher. *The Healing Arts: Exploring the Medical Ways of the World.* New York: Summit Books, 1987. Every culture has its own system of maintaining health. This lucid book draws the best from many and explains their relevance to contemporary Western medicine. It was given to me by Dr. Michael Fenster, who recommended it highly.

Enlightened Martial Arts

Dr. Masaaki Hatsumi. *Essence of Ninjutsu: The Nine Traditions*. Chicago: Contemporary Press, 1988. *Ninjutsu: History and Traditions*. Burbank, Calif.: Unique Publications, 1981. Only Hatsumi can express the feeling of ninjutsu from the grandmaster's viewpoint. One should go to the source while he is still living if you want to understand this complex art. None of his American interpreters are even close to the reality of his skill.

Taisen Deshimaru, Roshi. *The Zen Way to the Martial Arts*. New York: E. P. Dutton, Inc., 1982. Makes many oriental concepts accessible. It's required reading after Musashi for my students. Clearly states that bushido is a subset of butsudo. The samurai at his best.

Jou, Tsung Hwa. *The Tao of Tai-Chi Chuan: Way to Rejuvenation*. Piscataway, N.J.: The Tao Foundation or Charles E. Tuttle, Publishers, 1981. Reveals the history and relationship of tai chi to chi kung. Contains valuable information concerning centering, movement, and breathing exercises. Shows how the fundamentals of energy movement can be applied to any martial art.

Trevor Leggett. *Zen and the Ways*. Rutland, Vermont, and Tokyo: Charles E. Tuttle, 1987. Leggett has a number of books on the martial arts of Japan. He has been acknowledged by the Japanese government as a Westerner able to represent their thinking. His are the only translation of "warrior Zen" scrolls from the thirteenth century into English. He never loses sight of the practical implications of what he translates. Read.

Stephen P. Hayes. *The Ancient Art of Ninja Warfare: Combat, Espionage and Traditions*. Chicago: Contemporary, 1988. All of his work will eventually be collector items. He's the best American source of traditional training and historical information for the ninja enthusiast. He has entered the Mikkyo priesthood.

Strange Stuff that Won't Seem So Strange after a While

Dr. Rammamurti S. Mishras. *The Textbook of Yoga Psychology: A new translation and interpretation of Patanjali's Yoga Sutras for meaningful application in all modern psychologic disciplines.* New York: The Julian Press, 1963. Need I say more? Patanjali was the greatest psychologist in all of history. His exposition of the spiritual mental process is completely accurate and transcends cultural influence. He was a man for all times.

Gary Doore. *Shaman's Path: Healing, Personal Growth and Empowerment.* Boston and London: Shambhala, 1988. A very good collection of essays concerning modern applications of some very old ideas and principles.

Joseph Campbell, ed. *The Mythic Image.* Princeton, N.J.: Bollingen Series C, Princeton University Press, 1968. I wish I'd known about this book when I first started doing chi kung. Campbell has done an excellent job in popularizing and explaining the esoteric in religion across cultures.

Arthur Hastings. *With the Tongues of Men and Angels: A Study of Channeling.* Forth Worth, Texas: Hold, Rinehard and Winston, 1990. A more Christian perspective on channeling but presented with plenty of empirical back-up. Easy to read and comprehensive.

Felicitas D. Goodman. *Where the Spirits Ride the Wind: Trance Journeys and Other Ecstatic Experiences.* Bloomington and Indianapolis: Indiana University Press, 1990. Describes positions and rituals that invite rather interesting guests to come visit your body. Some of these women's groups make Robert Bly's bad boys look pretty harmless by comparison. I tried her stuff out and animal sensibility can be interesting.

Bruce A. Vance, Poet. *Dreamscape: Voyage in an alternate Reality.* Wheaton, Ill.: Quest Books, Theosophical Publishing House, 1989. The best book I've found concerning dreamwork. Very process- and experience-oriented and full of useful ideas that come from someone who has done what he is writing about. Let Vance be your guy in this tricky area.

Keep going. Keep playing. Study on this.

About the Author

GLENN J. MORRIS is an elected member of The World Martial Arts Hall of Fame. Dr. Morris was granted the title Oshihan by the Board of Directors of the Bun Bu-Ichi Zendo Budo/Bugei Remmei in 1991. In 1992 he was given the rank of Shichidan (seventh dan, black belt or nanaedan) in Bujinkan Ninpo. He has been ranked rokudan (sixth dan, black belt) in Nihon Karate Jujutsu and in 1990 passed the sword test for godan (fifth dan) in the legendary Togakure Ryu. He was personally given a Shidoshi's license in Bujinkan Ninpo by grandmaster Masaaki Hatsumi-Soke and 34th linear grandmaster of the oldest surviving school of combatic strategy in the world. Togakure Ryu ninjutsu has an unbroken lineage extending back to the eleventh century.

Following the directions for chi kung meditative practice recommended by Taoist scholars of 2500 years ago, in 1985 Dr. Morris survived what is commonly referred to as the arousal of the kundalini in yoga, and the greater kan and li by practitioners of Chinese esoteric meditation arts. After achieving these levels of mastery in traditional Asian systems of enlightenment, Glenn was able to replicate his experience for his own students using the scientific method to create a martial way appropriate for Americans (Hoshinroshiryu) but firmly based in the combat schools of China and Japan. He has also developed a less physical system for the not so athletically inclined as part of the Phoenix Whole Person Institute. Shidoshi Morris often demonstrates and presents as an instructor on the World Congress of Martial Arts teaching team.

Dr. Morris earned his bachelor's in General Arts and Science, master's in Speech at Penn State, and his Ph.D. in Communication at Wayne State. He completed a Doctor of Science in Psychology and Polemikology at Eurotechnical Research University and is Dean of General Academics for the recently founded Rockwell School of Applied Arts and Sciences degree programs for black belt-holding martial artists in traditional and eclectic systems at Hilo, Hawaii.

Dr. Morris has been a college professor and a psychological consultant to the Fortune 200 for most of his professional life. He has written and delivered empirically based strategical, motivational, and team-building programs to the automotive industry, school systems, grocery chains, power production corporations, the chemical industry, and retailers. He thinks of his martial arts accomplishments as simply milestones resulting from his hobbies. He is an independent representative of the National Educational Training Group of Michigan and consults with Mike Palmer and Robert Simpson Associates out of Flint, Michigan.

Dr. Morris has or has had professional memberships in the American Association for the Advancement of Science, Associations for Transpersonal and Humanistic Psychology, The Speech Communication Association, the International Society for the Study of Subtle Energy and Energy Medicine, Foundation for Shamanistic Research, Institute of Noetic Sciences, International Guild of Counselors and Therapists, and The National Guild of Hypnotists.